Henry J. Aaron
editor

The Future
of Academic
Medical Centers

BROOKINGS INSTITUTION PRESS
Washington, D.C.

Copyright © 2001 by

THE BROOKINGS INSTITUTION
1775 Massachusetts Avenue, N.W.
Washington, D.C. 20036
www.brookings.edu

Library of Congress Cataloging-in-Publication

The future of academic medical centers / Henry J. Aaron, editor.
  p. cm.
Includes index.
ISBN 0-8157-0236-1 (cloth) —ISBN 0-8157-0237-X (paper)
1. Teaching hospitals—United States—Finance. I. Aaron, Henry J.

RA975.T43 F88 2001   2001003398
362.1'1'0973—dc21

9 8 7 6 5 4 3 2 1

The paper used in this publication meets minimum requirements of the
American National Standard for Information Sciences—Permanence of
Paper for Printed Library Materials: ANSI Z39.48-1992.

Typeset in Sabon

Composition by AlphaWebTech
Mechanicsville, Maryland

Printing by R. R. Donnelley and Sons
Harrisonburg, Virginia

Foreword

The American academic medical center would rank high on any list of successful institutions. These centers lead the world in biomedical research. They offer top-quality treatment for the most serious and complicated illnesses. They turn out some of the best-trained physicians in the world. And they provide a disproportionate amount of care for the indigent and uninsured. For those reasons, the reports of acute financial distress emanating in recent years from some of the centers must be a source of profound concern to citizens and policymakers alike.

With financial support from the Agency for Healthcare Research and Quality of the U.S. Department of Health and Human Services, the Commonwealth Fund, and the Josiah Macy Jr. Foundation, Brookings convened a one-day conference of administrators, analysts, and congressional staff to assess the nature, extent, and depth of the financial problems besetting academic medical centers. The participants also considered what steps the centers themselves can take to improve their financial performance and what help public policy can provide.

The diagnosis is that a minority of medical centers will find it difficult to survive in an increasingly competitive and unforgiving environment in which private payers bargain aggressively and government programs curtail payments. But most centers can survive and prosper—the keys will be intelligent management that avoids repeating the extremely serious blunders of some medical center administrators during the 1990s and a framework of carefully designed public policies.

Kathleen Elliott Yinug assisted in arrangements for the conference and in the preparation of the manuscript; Ben Harris and Emily Tang provided research assistance; and Eileen Hughes edited the manuscript.

vii

The views expressed in this book are those of the authors and do not necessarily represent the position of the trustees, officers, or staff of the Brookings Institution.

MICHAEL H. ARMACOST
President, Brookings Institution

June 2001
Washington, D.C.

Contents

1. Introduction   1
    Henry J. Aaron

2. The Financial Health of Academic Medical
    Centers: An Elusive Subject   13
    Nancy M. Kane
    Comments by *Ralph Muller, James Reuter, and*
    Peter Van Etten
    General Discussion

3. Academic Medical Centers and
    the Economics of Innovation in Health Care   49
    James C. Robinson
    Comments by *David Blumenthal, Spencer Foreman, and*
    Edward Miller
    General Discussion

4. Politically Feasible and Practical Public Policies
    to Help Academic Medical Centers   75
    Lawrence S. Lewin
    Comments by *Robert Dickler, Kenneth I. Shine, and*
    Gail Wilensky
    General Discussion

Contributors   103

Index   105

CHAPTER ONE

Introduction

Henry J. Aaron

D epending on whom you talk to, U.S. academic medical centers are in
a financial crisis that threatens their viability or they are going through
a market shakeup that is punishing them for past financial practices. Clearly,
many of the nation's academic medical centers are financially stressed.
What is unclear is how extensive the problem is and what public policy
can do about it. Conditions seem to have improved over the past year, but
it is also unclear whether the improvement is sufficient to save the minority of seriously troubled institutions.

What Is an Academic Medical Center?

An academic medical center (AMC) consists of three related enterprises: a
medical school that trains physicians; research activities involving laboratory science, clinical investigation, or both; and a system for delivering
health care services that may include one or more hospitals, satellite clinics, and a physician practice plan. Those functions may be organized in
many ways. In many—perhaps most—cases, a single organization owns
and operates all three, but there are numerous exceptions. George Washington University, for example, sold controlling interest in its hospital to a
for-profit hospital chain. Harvard University runs no clinical practice and
owns no hospital; instead, it places its students in various hospitals in
Boston.

Academic medical centers follow many patterns. As the CEO of one
center put it: "If you have seen one academic medical center, you have
seen one academic medical center." Some urban AMCs operate in competitive markets that have too many beds, and many confront large man-

aged care organizations with close to sole purchasing power. On the other hand, some specialty hospitals may enjoy some market power, as do medical center hospitals in small communities where the competition is geographically distant.

The linking of education, research, and service delivery that is typical of the U.S. academic medical center provides important benefits to each function. After the first two years of classroom instruction, budding medical practitioners embark on a series of clinical rotations. Newly minted MDs may pursue postgraduate education that includes an internship, a residency, and a subspecialty fellowship. Those who are attracted to laboratory research go through a similar apprenticeship, usually under the guidance of a senior mentor.

Linking functions also raises the quality of health services provided by teaching hospitals, whose medical superiority rests in some measure on the presence of low-paid junior staff, undergraduate interns, and graduate student residents. Recognizing the superior services made possible by medical students, Medicare pays about $6 billion a year extra to teaching hospitals. But no one knows how to measure or value the difference in quality, which is the first step in determining whether that payment represents a reasonable price. As a result, the extra payment is based on cost.

It can be said, without discounting the role of the nation's wealth and size, that linking teaching, research, and service delivery by talented, relatively inexpensive staff has contributed greatly to the preeminence of U.S. medical science in the latter half of the twentieth century (see figure 1-1).

The Financial History of the Academic Medical Center

With the exception of tuition and fees, which never have accounted for a large share of medical school income, the mix of revenues flowing to medical schools changed dramatically from 1955 to 1997 (see figure 1-2).

Following World War II, many hospitals in the United States were expanded or built with the help of federal subsidies. Tax-exempt bonds continue to support hospital construction today. As hospitals were being built, however, advances in medical technology caused the average length of a hospital stay to decline steadily—by about one-quarter over the past 25 years.

Other developments increased the use of hospitals. Medical advances lengthened the menu of hospital-based services. Teaching hospitals benefited because the price of new technology typically is set high and comes

Figure 1-1. *Nobel Prizes in Medicine*

Number of prizes

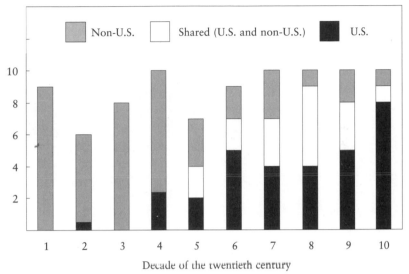

Decade of the twentieth century

down more slowly than costs. The growth of private and then public insurance also increased hospital use by enabling more people to afford it. Before the early 1990s, fee-for-service reimbursement under private insurance and cost-based reimbursement under public insurance enabled hospitals to cover all their costs, variable and fixed. In fact, weak limits on reimbursable costs meant that hospitals connected to academic medical centers became cash cows, generating surpluses that could be used to increase faculty and expand research programs.

The number of hospital beds peaked in 1983, just two years after hospital occupancy rates began a decline that has been interrupted only briefly in the period since (figure 1-3). Despite the steady, if slow, drop in the number of hospital beds, occupancy rates have continued to fall. New technology has enabled physicians to provide services in outpatient clinics or their offices that once required hospital admission. And, especially since the early 1990s, managed care organizations, which hold hospitalization rates dramatically below those of other payers, have come to serve an increasing portion of the population.

Although medical school faculties have treated patients for a long time, their practices contributed little to medical school revenues until the 1960s, when medical school deans and university presidents recognized that phy-

Figure 1-2. *Sources of Medical School Revenues, Selected Years*

Percent of total revenue

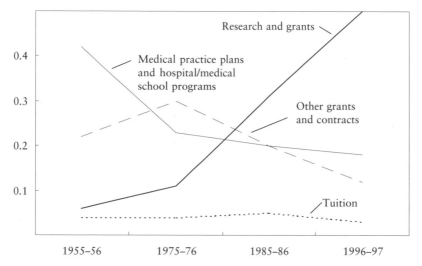

sician practice plans and hospital revenues could generate sizable surpluses. Those surpluses, in turn, could be used to support faculty expansion and research and other activities. Various medical services currently account for roughly half of medical school revenues and about 90 percent of hospital revenues. Because the surpluses generated by practice plans and hospitals are the difference between very large costs and very large revenues, even small adjustments in those gross flows have enormous significance.

What Is the Problem?

All but one of the forces that made academic medical centers a remarkably good business have been reversed. The seeming exception has been federal spending on health research and training, which jumped 64 percent in constant dollars between 1990 and 2000 and is expected to continue to rise during the first decade of the new century. But federal grants can be a mixed blessing. AMCs complain that reimbursement for research fails to cover all their indirect costs and that the federal cap on reimbursement for direct salary costs is well below actual salaries. Some hospital administrators report that for every $100 in research grants, they must raise roughly $10 from private donations or other sources to sustain their research programs.

Figure 1-3.   *Hospital Beds and Occupancy Rates, 1978–96*

Beds (thousands)   Occupancy rate (percent)

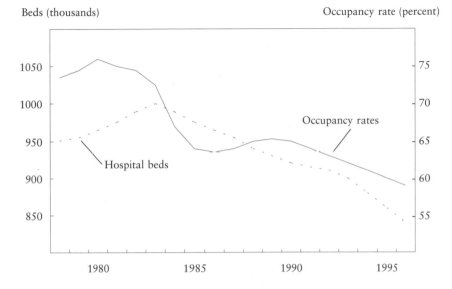

All other major sources of hospital revenue (figure 1-4) have come under increasingly strict control. In 1983, Congress amended the rules for payment of Medicare inpatient hospital services. Instead of reimbursing hospitals for actual costs, the Health Care Financing Administration (renamed Centers for Medicare and Medicaid Services in June 2001) established prospective payments related to patient diagnosis on admission. The initial payments and annual increases more than covered costs attributed to Medicare patients. But, in 1997, as part of the Balanced Budget Act, Congress scaled back payments by about 10 percent for the succeeding four years. There is some dispute about whether the cuts merely reduced margins or were so severe that Medicare payments ceased to cover costs of Medicare patients. Congress twice "gave back" some of those cuts—in 1999 and 2000.

At the same time, the states increasingly have shifted to contracts with managed care organizations to serve the Medicaid population. The 1997 legislation also mandated prospective payment for outpatient services. In addition, private insurance, which once paid what hospitals charged, was replaced by negotiated contracts with managed care organizations. Hospitals entered into such contracts mistakenly expecting Medicare payments to remain at pre-1997 levels.

As occupancy rates fell, hospitals' power to resist managed care weakened. Managed care organizations could offer any price over marginal

Figure 1-4. *Composition of Hospital Revenues, 1998*

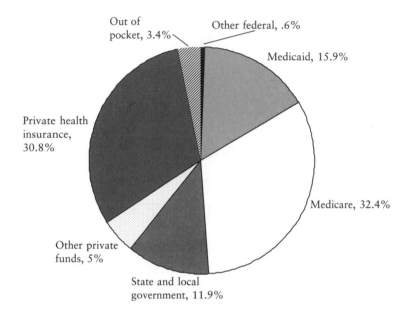

cost to underused facilities with many empty beds; if a hospital in a competitive market refused an offer, the organization could shop elsewhere. Hospitals accepted the deals but found that overhead charges rested on a smaller and smaller base, and for many hospitals, operating margins narrowed and became negative. Hospitals responded by canceling some contracts in 1999 and 2000 and insisting on higher fees.

Finally, the proportion of the population with private health insurance fell 5 percentage points between 1987 and 1993. Although the drop in private coverage was partly offset by increases in Medicaid and Medicare, the share of the population without insurance—and therefore dependent on charity care—grew. After 1993, private insurance coverage leveled off, but the share of people with employer-sponsored insurance rose 5 percentage points by 1998. The move from individual to group coverage shifted demand from weak to strong bargainers.

The Consequences

Academic medical centers and other hospitals responded to the worsening financial environment in various ways. A few tried to cut costs by reducing staff and closing beds, but most added to staff—faculty increased 41 percent during the 1990s. Many centers tried to increase occupancy rates by underbidding competitors. To generate revenue and channel more cases to the parent hospital, others opened satellite primary care clinics or purchased physician practices. Many hospitals merged as their managers sought economies of scale and increased market power.

While some hospital executives responded to the new sensitivity to prices with imagination and astuteness, others blundered. Perhaps the most egregious case involved the Allegheny Health, Education, and Research Foundation. Between 1986 and 1997, it grew by acquisition and merger from a single hospital with 740 beds and revenues of $195 million to a consortium of 14 hospitals operating throughout Pennsylvania with 4,601 beds and revenues of $2.2 billion. The organization also amassed $1.3 billion in debt and 65,000 creditors. In 1998 it declared bankruptcy.

That medical bankruptcy, the largest in history, led bond-rating agencies to reassess academic medical centers. By early 1999, the agencies had either downgraded the bonds of or projected a negative outlook for many AMCs, including Harvard's CareGroup, Johns Hopkins, the University of Pennsylvania, Washington University, Baylor University, and Duke University. Even worse, some hospitals found it impossible to buy bond insurance, which they need to float new issues at reasonable cost.

A year before the Allegheny debacle, a careful study reported that from 1986 through 1994, hospitals that merged began with higher revenues and costs but that their costs and revenues rose less rapidly than those of stand-alone hospitals. The authors concluded that mergers and alliances were a promising way to bring down costs. Yet, just two years later, in the wake of the Allegheny collapse, a review of nearly half of 750 hospital mergers and alliances formed between 1993 through 1997 found that few had achieved intended economic advantages. Another study confirmed that partners in health alliances had slightly higher revenues per bed and per discharge but that they also had higher costs. Then, a much-heralded alliance between the University of California at San Francisco and Stanford University that had promised to lower costs and cut staff instead raised costs and added 1,700 positions. The alliance was dissolved, and heads rolled.

Part of the increased efficiency from mergers comes from consolidating functions and firing people, which are particularly troublesome undertakings at a university with tenured faculty and staff. Fewer problems arise when nonprofit AMC hospitals are acquired by investor-owned chains. A study of three such mergers found no adverse effects on teaching, research, or indigent care.

One strategy for improving financial viability—the purchase of physician practices—was pursued with particular vigor and at high cost at the University of Pennsylvania. The medical center was to provide the physicians with certain services, and the physicians were expected to refer patients to the medical center in return. But university administrators failed to foresee that transferring a lot of cash to middle-aged practitioners and reducing their incremental compensation for seeing more patients would reduce work effort. In addition, the physicians put the interests of their patients above those of the hospital administrators by continuing to refer patients on the basis of a hospital's quality and proximity to the patients or to themselves.

Partly because of those errors, the Pennsylvania medical center lost $180 million in 1999 and its highly esteemed dean joined the lengthy list of academic medical center CEOs who have resigned following large losses.

What It Means and What Policymakers Should Do

Several academic medical centers are in deep trouble. But whether AMCs as a group are in deep trouble is much less certain. It is difficult, also, to determine how much of the trouble results from poor administration and ill-considered business decisions and how much from an increasingly unforgiving business environment.

Fragmentary evidence suggests that the financial problems of academic medical centers are serious and widespread. Other evidence suggests that serious problems exist only in a few centers. Several facts—that there is a glut of hospital beds, that the market power of managed care organizations is growing, and that since 1977 payments under Medicare have been reduced—all signal a deterioration in the financial condition of hospitals in general and AMCs in particular. Downgrades by bond-rating organizations and the huge losses reported by many academic medical centers testify to genuine financial distress. Even such strong organizations as the Partners Healthcare System in Boston (Massachusetts General Hospital and Peter Bent Brigham Hospital) report declining margins, which may force them to dip into their endowment and reserves, or worse. Faced with such downward trends, academic medical centers seem to differ only in when they will go into the red.

Nevertheless, some analysts strongly dispute the allegations that AMCs are in trouble. An article published in 1999 in the journal *Health Affairs* pointed out that the proportion of academic health centers with negative operating margins fell between 1989 and 1995 from 35 percent to 19 percent. Between 1993 and 1997 several other financial measures—cash reserves on hand, return on equity, and long-term debt/equity ratios—all improved for hospitals in and outside academic medical centers. Some critics said that the data in the article preceded the 1997 Balanced Budget Act, which reduced both Medicare and Medicaid payments. Another study, sponsored by the American Hospital Association, estimated that Medicare payments failed to cover hospital costs starting in 1999 and that, even allowing for legislation enacted in 1999, the shortfall will increase.

On the other hand, MedPac, a congressionally mandated commission that oversees Medicare, concluded in 1999 that "hospitals . . . appear to be in good financial shape overall" and in 2000 that "there is little evidence that policy changes enacted in the Balanced Budget Act have harmed beneficiaries' access to care." My own analysis of data for 1994–98, supplied by the Association of American Medical Colleges, found little evidence that the finances of academic medical center hospitals deteriorated over that period. And there is some evidence that conditions improved somewhat during 1999.

Nancy Kane addresses these questions in her chapter in this volume. Because each academic medical center is somewhat idiosyncratic and no uniform accounting conventions exist, forming generalizations is extremely difficult. She finds that a minority of medical centers seems to be in deep trouble, while the remainder face a difficult environment but probably will survive.

All AMCs must decide what their "business plan" should be. They deliver high-quality services in an increasingly cost-conscious market. They compete against community hospitals that provide generally less sophisticated services at lower average cost. In recent years, many AMCs have adopted ill-considered business strategies and have paid a high price for doing so. In his chapter, James Robinson addresses the question of how medical centers should manage their affairs in order to capitalize on their unique advantage as centers of medical innovation and research.

The Policymaker's Problem and Some Solutions

The problem for policymakers is that the available facts are consistent with two different stories. The first is that the financial environment of AMCs has turned hostile, that the failing hospitals and those with large losses have been the canaries in the coal mine, and that other serious problems will follow. Academic medical centers, it is argued, cannot continue to perform all of their traditional functions without help; the unstated premise is that policy should be changed to help them.

The second story is that for decades academic medicine lived a life of financial privilege, free from the usual market pressures. It acquired loose financial habits that bring swift punishment in the new Darwinian economy. Centers with strong faculties face particular challenges because it is hard to compel people with many career options to sacrifice their quality of life—by seeing more patients or ordering fewer tests—simply to improve the medical center's bottom line. And the evidence that AMCs as a group are financially threatened remains equivocal, at best.

The one almost universally accepted fact is that the United States still has way too many hospital beds. Furthermore, demand for those beds is likely to continue to decline because of new drugs and other medical advances. Until some hospitals close—and that probably includes some academic medical centers—excess capacity and cutthroat pricing will be inescapable. Furthermore, AMCs face a host of new challenges, among them the need to modify medical education and the high capital costs of converting the traditional health care system based on personal communication and paper records to the new world of modern information technology.

On the way to a new equilibrium, many hospitals doubtless will suffer considerable financial distress. There is no guarantee that the right hospitals will fail. Closing hospitals can seriously disrupt the economic life of communities, which will fight ferociously to keep them open. The charitable or religious organizations that run many hospitals may accept low returns or losses indefinitely to provide emergency and primary care to urban uninsured populations. In rural areas, a hospital closure can cut people off from medical services entirely.

As for the functions now joined in academic medical centers—medical research, teaching, and patient care—no one knows whether there are other equally effective ways to perform them. The achievements of U.S. biomedical research, high standards of care, and superior medical education may suffer as hospitals downsize. However, the cost of the error of providing too much help to medical centers and the cost of the error of providing too little are not equal. If too much help is given, money will be wasted. If too little is given, important research and teaching institutions could suffer great damage. That said, it is not clear what policymakers can do to spare AMCs the financial suffering that the hospital sector as a whole will have to experience.

At present, federal policymakers can take two actions that can directly help academic medical centers—reform the Medicare payment system and reform the system for payment of indirect research costs. Only the first is significant. Medicare makes two payments to teaching hospitals—direct payments to offset added salary costs and indirect payments to offset the extra costs, such as those for additional tests, incurred in teaching hospitals. Because of econometric errors, Medicare initially set the indirect payments too high. Congress subsequently has been lowering them, but they still are about $1.5 billion higher than is justifiable. Those overgenerous payments have encouraged an increase in the number of residents from 60,000 to about 100,000; increasing the assistance would be hard to defend. If Congress wishes to support medical education, the program should be financed through general revenues, not Medicare.

The cumulative effect of the Balanced Budget Act of 1997 (as modified by the Balanced Budget Refinement Act of 1999) will be to lower academic hospital revenues about 3 percent in 2002. The cuts affect all hospitals, but not equally. Rescinding some of the cuts would distribute aid among all hospitals and slow the necessary process of downsizing. The second reform involves reimbursements to universities for indirect research costs, currently about $2 billion annually. Replacing the elaborate and expensive cost-accounting approach would free up resources that could be applied to research costs.

Beyond these modest steps, it is hard to make a persuasive case that academic medical centers as a group merit general financial assistance. Even if one could make that case, it is hard to conceive of politically sustainable methods of channeling aid to them. New methods of assistance to AMCs will have to be found if some of the institutions are to be spared the rigors of the new health care marketplace. In his chapter, Lawrence Lewin describes a number of measures that policymakers in Washington can take and that medical centers can implement to help meet the new educational and information challenges they face.

CHAPTER TWO

The Financial Health of Academic Medical Centers: An Elusive Subject

Nancy M. Kane

From 1999 through 2000, headlines across the country proclaimed the financial woes of academic medical centers in Chicago, San Francisco, Columbus, Philadelphia, Boston, New York, and Washington, D.C., warning of the damage from cutbacks in Medicare, reductions in managed care revenues, and competition from large community hospitals.[1] Those well-publicized crises stimulated calls for public policy interventions ranging from a freeze on cuts instituted by the Balanced Budget Act of 1997 (BBA) to establishment of special trust funds to pay for the social missions of AMCs, financed by all payers or by general tax revenues.[2] Despite the warnings, it may well be short-sighted to provide additional financial advantages to an industry that already has substantial advantages and in which financial crises have appeared over only the last two years.

In November 2000, the bond-rating agency Standard & Poor's (S&P) issued a report on academic medical centers that noted that they have fundamental strengths, including broad regional market penetration, strong regional and sometimes national reputations, and great financial flexibility.[3] Advantages accruing to many AMCs include special state and federal subsidies, strong fund-raising capabilities, and dominance in the market for specialized services, which permits them to charge premium prices.

---

1. See, for instance, Marquis (2000); Powers (2000); Casey (1999); Knox and Zitner (1999); and Herbert (1999).

2. Blumenthal and Thier (1998).

3. Rodgers, Zuckerman, and Goode (2000).

According to the S&P report, most AMCs still enjoy financial ratings of A or higher, in part because of their historically strong financial performance before 1998. S&P concluded that financial pressures on AMCs have increased lately but that some "have managed not only to survive but also prosper."

In this chapter, I try to clarify the financial situation of a sample of AMCs and through that process to provide insight into what is and is not known about the recent financial performance of AMCs in general. I identify and quantify some of the sources of financial stress that AMCs experienced in 1998 and 1999; I also comment on the need for and the possible nature of public interventions on behalf of AMCs.

Analytic Challenges in Determining the Financial Health of AMCs

Financial analysis of AMCs faces four major challenges: AMCs are complex entities; they employ disparate financial reporting practices; sufficient data on their financial performance are hard to obtain; and data tend to be released only after considerable delay.

Complexity of AMCs

AMCs typically include a medical school, its closely affiliated clinical facilities, and faculty practice plans.[4] Those components may be owned and governed by a single organization, or each component may be separately owned and governed. Sometimes the single owner is a university, although universities increasingly have spun off their AMCs into independent and autonomous operating units. Closely affiliated clinical facilities may include several community hospitals, networks of community physicians, and providers of home care, rehabilitation, and skilled nursing services. Such diverse businesses as health insurance companies, real estate firms, biotechnology ventures, sports training facilities, and assisted living and retirement communities also are controlled, managed, or otherwise supported by AMCs.

Figure 2-1a provides an overview of the components of CareGroup, a Boston AMC with $1.8 billion in assets in 1999. CareGroup's constellation of roughly twenty affiliates is relatively simple; the most complex

4. Rodgers, Zuckerman, and Goode (2000, p. 330).

unit in my sample had nearly fifty affiliates. CareGroup, a major teaching hospital of Harvard Medical School but separately owned and governed, consists of a parent organization; one major teaching hospital, Beth Israel Deaconess Medical Center (BIDMC); five other community/specialty hospitals; each hospital's subsidiaries (owned physician practices, a hospice, a property management company, and a management company); and seven other related entities, including faculty practice plans, a provider service network (contracting organization), a management services organization, two research groups, the Mind-Body Institute, and a wellness and fitness center (figure 2-1b). While other AMCs may have different businesses and services in their related entities, they resemble CareGroup in their complexity and range of clinical and nonclinical undertakings. Differences among AMCs may be as great as similarities in both function and form.

Financial Reporting Practices

AMCs differ in how they report their financial relationships with affiliates and how they classify key financial elements. The AMC may take a *minimalist* approach, including financial results of only the operating unit of the major teaching hospital. That approach corresponds most directly with the entity reporting seen in Medicare cost reports and the Internal Revenue Service's Form 990, described later. State agencies that maintain audited financial information about their hospitals also generally collect data on single hospitals.

An *intermediate* reporting option is to consolidate the financial results of all affiliates that share an obligation to repay specific issues of long-term debt; those affiliates constitute an "obligated group." Creditors commonly request such reporting. However, one of the reasons for the lack of prior warning of the bankruptcy of Allegheny Health, Education, and Research Foundation was that the overall picture was never presented. Creditors were given the financial results of five different obligated groups, and the impact of one group on another was not disclosed.[5]

The most *comprehensive* approach is to consolidate the financial results of every affiliate that is at least 50 percent controlled by the parent or by any parent-controlled subsidiary. That reporting method, which provides an overview of all of the AMC's components, permits detailed assessment of the whole but reveals less about the performance of each part.

5. Burns, Cacciamani, Clement, and Aquino (2000).

Figure 2-1a. *Components of CareGroup*[a]

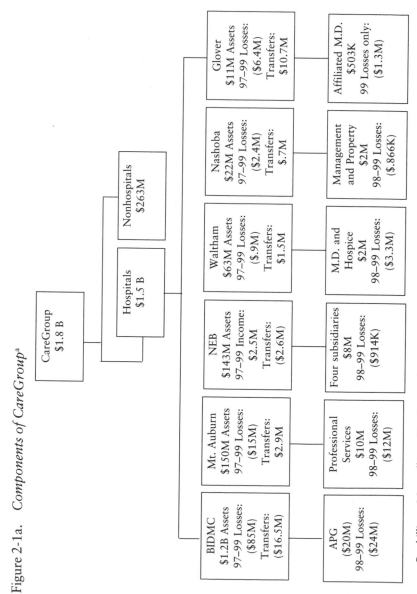

Figure 2-1b. *CareGroup's Nonhospital Subsidiaries*

Nonhospital Subsidiaries
$263M

CareGroup Parent
$168M
97–99 Losses: ($8.7M)
97–99 Transfers: $12.1M

HMFP
$31M
97–99 Income: $9.3M
97–99 Transfers: $2.5M

Picker Institute
97–99 Losses: ($1.9M)
97–99 Transfers: $0

MSO
98–99 Losses: ($199K)
97–99 Transfers: $1.5M

Academic Research Group
$11M
97–99 Income: $1.5M
97–99 Transfers: $2.7M

Wellness and Fitness Center
$33M
97–99 Losses: ($3.3M)
97–99 Transfers: $2M

Mind-Body Institute
$5M
97–99 Income: $1.2M
97–99 Transfers: $0

PSN
$250K
97–99 Losses: $0
97–99 Transfers: $250K

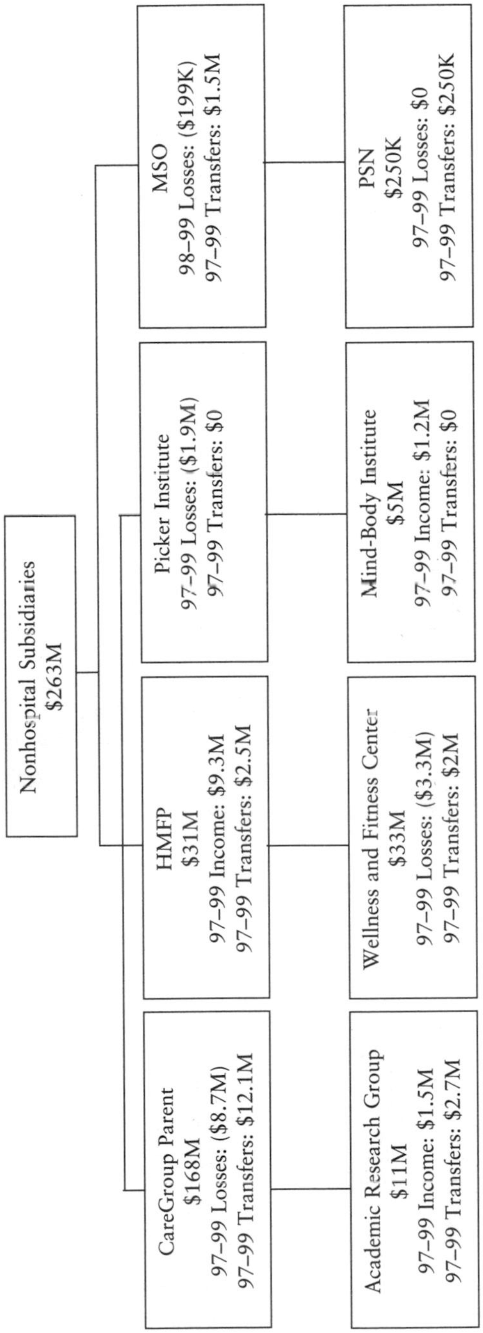

Supplemental information on component businesses may be disclosed in the comprehensive financial report. Again, primarily creditors request comprehensive entity data. There also are gradations in reporting style between the minimalist, intermediate, and comprehensive approaches.

The reporting format of one AMC may differ greatly from that of another, making comparison of their financial performance difficult and potentially misleading. Even within a single AMC, the financial condition of components may differ greatly. For instance, the Mary Hitchcock Medical Center (MHMC) at Dartmouth University reported a total margin of 9.5 percent and an operating margin of 1.9 percent in 1999. However, the Mary Hitchcock obligated group (which includes MHMC, the Hitchcock Clinic, and two community hospitals) reported a total margin of 5 percent and an operating margin of only .5 percent—marginally profitable but less than MHMC alone. The Hospital of the University of Pennsylvania reported a dismal 1999 operating margin of *minus* 11 percent, while the operating margin of its obligated group was a quite respectable 9 percent.

Figure 2-2 provides an overview of the various ways that the financial results of AMC affiliates may be reflected on the financial statements of the AMC core (assuming that the AMC core includes only the major teaching hospital and perhaps the medical school). In the first block from the core are affiliates that are at least 50 percent owned or controlled by the core AMC (such as BIDMC's owned physician practice, APG, in figure 2-1a). They are consolidated with the core AMC, and balance sheets and income statements for both are summed together and reported as one. In the second block are affiliates that may be independent in terms of board and management control of resources but that have contractually obligated themselves to meet debt service requirements for a common debt issue; those affiliates would constitute an entity within an obligated group. In the third block are unconsolidated affiliates; they may be controlled by a parent corporation that also controls the AMC, may buy and sell services to the core AMC, and may exchange cash and other assets with the core AMC. Their financial statements, however, are not consolidated with those of the AMC. Transfers and buying/selling transactions between unconsolidated affiliates and the core AMC are disclosed in the core AMC's footnotes to its financial statement. In the outer block are equity investment ventures over which the core AMC has significant influence but not control, generally having less than 50 percent ownership. The AMC balance sheet carries the equity investment at cost, net of gains and losses,

Figure 2-2. *AMC Financial Reporting Categories*

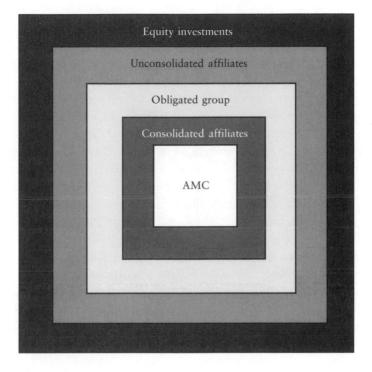

and the AMC's share of gains and losses is reported on the AMC income statement.

How affiliates are recognized within the reporting entity can make a great difference in an outsider's understanding of an institution's financial health. For instance, the University of Pittsburgh Medical Center (UPMC) is one of the five AMCs in my sample for which the financial information was consolidated without supplemental disclosure of the performance of the various entities within the AMC. Other public information revealed that over the period 1997–99, the hospital division of UPMC earned cumulative operating profits of roughly $88 million; losses on the nonhospital divisions—physicians ($180 million operating loss), insurance ($60 million operating loss), and diversified ventures ($5 million operating loss)—resulted in systemwide operating losses throughout the period.[6]

6. Gaynor (2000).

AMC financial reports differ not only in how they consolidate entities but also in how they classify such key financial elements as investment income (interest, dividends, and realized gains on marketable securities); unrealized gains and losses; and assets, including cash and marketable securities whose uses are restricted. Investment income was a primary source of positive margins for many AMCs in the late 1990s; traditionally such income was separated from operating income and called "nonoperating revenue" on the income statement.[7] Operating income was defined as net income earned by the entity from the provision of services central to its mission, such as patient care, teaching, and research. In recent years, however, many hospitals, including many AMCs, have reported investment income as part of operating revenues and income, thus masking their operating results. Unrealized gains and losses are not supposed to be reported as part of income, but rather as part of other changes in net assets (equity).[8] However, some AMCs have reported unrealized gains as revenues, in fact as operating revenues, again masking the actual results from operations, defined above. When such information is properly disclosed in footnotes, the analyst can remove investment income from operating income; I have made those adjustments for the AMCs in my sample.

Finally, the nature of the restrictions on the use of an AMC's cash and marketable securities may not be disclosed. Some limitations can be undone by action of the board of directors. Others are imposed by contracts with outside creditors or regulators and cannot be undone without breaching the contract. Still others are stipulated by donors; in such cases the donor must be reimbursed if the funds are not used as stipulated. Understanding the nature of limitations on cash and marketable securities is necessary to calculate "days of cash on hand," a ratio that indicates how liquid an AMC is (discussed later). Many AMCs, though they lost money on operations in 1998 and 1999, had accumulated significant cash reserves through profits and cash flows of prior years. Proper disclosure of the availability of cash to meet short-term operating or financial needs is critical to assessing the financial condition of an AMC. Again, that reporting issue generally can be resolved by the analyst with information provided in footnotes to audited financial statements.

7. By 1999, some AMCs had invested as much as 64 percent of their investment portfolio in equities; the average for my sample was 40 percent, with a range of 0 percent to 64 percent. Rating agencies view that trend as a source of concern, given the volatility of the stock market. See, for instance, Arrick, Rodgers, and Gigante (2000).

8. American Institute of Certified Public Accountants (1998).

Availability of Comprehensive Financial Data

There are four major sources of financial information about AMCs and other hospitals in the United States.

Medicare Cost Reports (MCR) are publicly available and provide information on every hospital entity that has a Medicare contract, a description that includes most hospitals. The MCR provides the information used to develop several of the publicly available commercial databases on hospital financial performance. However, MCRs do not provide sufficient detail, either in the balance sheet or the income statement, to permit adjustment of differences in reporting practices among hospitals. They do not include footnotes, a vital source of information about affiliates, marketable securities, commitments and contingencies, and the way that investment income and unrealized gains are categorized in the reports. They include only the hospital entity, not affiliates.[9]

Self-reported surveys by the American Hospital Association (AHA) and the American Association of Medical Colleges (AAMC) are conducted regularly. The data are not audited by external objective parties, and information on individual hospitals generally is not available to the public. Results often are reported to the public as averages rather than as the distribution of values for all hospitals. As with the MCR, the focus of the surveys tends to be the hospital entity alone.

IRS Form 990 is the annual report to the Internal Revenue Service required of all charitable institutions. The reports are available to the public on request, and many organizations have put their recent filings on a website (www.guidestar.org). The data consist of an income statement and a balance sheet, with numerous disclosures presented in a nonstandardized series of attachments. The reports may contain much or little detail, and the elements do not always correspond to those reported in the MCR or audited financial statements. The reporting entity is the organization with the tax identification number, generally a single hospital or hospital affiliate. The form contains a schedule with information on the names, assets, recent income, and tax-exempt status of all affiliated organizations.

Audited financial statements are produced by most business entities, including all private nonprofit hospitals and most publicly owned hospitals. They contain more detail than do other sources of data, including three financial statements plus footnote disclosures that may run ten to

9. More details on the shortfalls of the MCR for financial reporting purposes are described in Kane and Magnus (2001).

fifteen pages, and they observe generally accepted accounting principles, introducing at least some measure of uniformity in reporting. Audited financial statements are considered the gold standard for financial reporting by the AHA and the Healthcare Financial Management Association.[10]

Timeliness of Financial Reporting

One of the greatest shortcomings of hospital financial reviews based on publicly available data is the lag between the end of a hospital's fiscal year and the date of release of financial data. The Health Care Financing Administration (HCFA) does not release the public MCR data until roughly two years after the close of the hospital's fiscal year; IRS 990 forms are available only ten months to two years after the end of the fiscal year to which they refer. Annual surveys by the AHA or the AAMC are not released to the public on a timely basis either; for instance, the AAMC Data Book for the year 2000 provided financial data for 1997.

The only relatively timely source of financial data is audited financial statements, which normally are completed within three months after the close of the fiscal year. Their public release, however, may be much slower, and hospitals in some states refuse to release audited financial statements to the public. There is no central national repository of audited financial statements for hospitals. Roughly half the states require hospitals to provide audited statements to a state agency that releases the data to the public, and some of those states have deadlines that are within six months of the close of the fiscal year. Recent Securities and Exchange Commission regulations require annual public filing of audited financial statements to municipal repositories by nonprofit hospitals that have issued tax-exempt debt since 1996, but the lag in filing can be as long as one year.

This analysis uses audited financial statements from either municipal repositories or state agencies that collect audited financial statements.[11] At the time this chapter was written, from December 2000 to January 2001, fiscal year 2000 data were not publicly available for most of the sample.

---

10. American Hospital Association (1990); also the Healthcare Financial Management Association (1994).

11. Roughly twenty-two to twenty-five states require hospitals to file audited financial statements and release them to the public. See Kane and Magnus (2001).

Sample of AMCs Selected for Analysis

Fifteen AMCs are included in the results shown here (for summary information, see table 2-1). Ten of them represent just the teaching hospital and one or two minor subsidiaries at most, on the minimalist end of the continuum for entity options.[12] The eleventh AMC is an obligated group of six consolidated affiliate hospitals;[13] AMCs twelve through fifteen report as comprehensive entities including not only hospitals but also insurance companies, physician practices, home care and long-term care organizations, and commercial ventures.[14] The AMCs chosen were a convenience sample based on availability of data for the three years from 1997 through 1999.

The sample average for number of beds is only 8 percent greater than the Council of Teaching Hospitals (COTH) average, but averages for admissions (43 percent greater), outpatient visits (79 percent greater), and full-time employees (90 percent greater) are significantly greater than the COTH averages, while the occupancy rate (68 percent) is slightly below. The sample overrepresents the Northeast, underrepresents the South and West, and fairly represents the Midwest. Only two publicly owned AMCs are in the sample (13 percent, below the 22 percent in the COTH group), and there are no investor-owned AMCs, compared with 3 percent in the COTH group. The significance of these variations is unclear. The AAMC does not provide extensive or current financial data about the COTH members. Table 2-2 suggests that the sample hospitals were performing roughly at the average COTH operating and total margins in 1997 but that they fell far below the COTH average in 1998.

While conclusions can only be tentative given the limited COTH data available, the sample appears to represent hospitals whose service vol-

12. The ten minimalist entities are Beth Israel Deaconess Medical Center, Brigham & Women's Hospital, Charleston Area Medical Center, Hospital of the University of Pennsylvania, Mary Hitchcock Medical Center, Massachusetts General Hospital, Rhode Island Hospital, Rush–Presbyterian–St. Luke's Medical Center, University of Illinois at Chicago, and University of Colorado Hospital.

13. Detroit Medical Center includes in the obligated group the following hospitals: Detroit Receiving Hospital and University Health Center, Children's Hospital of Michigan, Harper-Hutzel Hospital, Huron Valley–Sinai Hospital, Rehabilitation Institute of Michigan, and Sinai-Grace Hospital.

14. The four comprehensive entities include Clarian Health Partners (six consolidated affiliates), Shands (eleven consolidated affiliates), Duke University Health System (eight consolidated affiliates), and University of Pittsburg Medical Center (four major divisions, one of which includes thirteen hospitals).

Table 2-1. *Comparison of Sample to COTH Data*[a]

	Council of Teaching Hospitals (COTH)	Sample
Average		
Beds	491	529
Admissions	20,789	29,791
Outpatient visits	301,766	539,526
Full-time equivalent employees	2,896	5,527
Occupancy	72 percent	68 percent
Location		
Northeast	36 percent	47 percent
South	27 percent	20 percent
Midwest	26 percent	27 percent
West	11 percent	7 percent
Ownership		
Public	22 percent	13 percent
Private nonprofit	75 percent	87 percent
Investor-owned	3 percent	0 percent
Number of observations	277	15

Source: COTH data, *The AAMC Data Book, 2000* (Washington: Association of American Medical Colleges). Sample data, *AHA Guide to the Health Care Field*, 1999–2000 (Chicago).

[a]For multihospital entities, the values of only the major teaching hospital(s) are included in the comparison data.

ume is much higher than the COTH average but whose financial performance was significantly worse in 1998 than that of the average AMC. The ownership bias is not likely to be the cause of the difference in performance (public hospitals would not be expected to do better than private nonprofits), but the overrepresentation of the Northeast may be a factor. Compared with those in the South, hospitals in the Northeast experience higher managed care penetration and slower population

Table 2-2. *Comparisons of Sample and COTH Operating and Total Margins*[a]

Data	1997	1998
	Average operating margin	
COTH	1.58 percent	1.90 percent
Sample	1.19 percent	−3.20 percent
	Average total margin	
COTH	4.42 percent	3.30 percent
Sample	4.49 percent	1.39 percent

Source: 1997 data are from *The AAMC Data Book, 2000* (Washington: Association of American Medical Colleges). 1998 data are from *COTH Reports* (Washington: Association of American Medical Colleges).

[a]Operating margins exclude investment income; total margins include investment income in both the numerator and the denominator.

growth (potentially increasing competition), which could contribute to poorer financial outcomes.

Findings

Because the 1997–99 period affected AMCs quite differently, I present the financial results as a distribution of values rather than averages. Hospital boards, policymakers, and the public tend to focus on operating profits as the primary evidence of financial health or distress. I grouped the fifteen hospitals into high-performance (top quartile), medium-performance (middle 50 percent), and low-performance (bottom quartile) groups on the basis of their operating margins—(revenues minus expenses)/revenues, excluding investment income from revenues—from 1997 through 1999 (figure 2-3). While most hospitals did not remain in the same quartile each year, some stayed in the top or bottom quartiles in at least two of the three years. Four hospitals stayed in the bottom quartile for at least two of three years (the low-performance group), and four hospitals stayed in the top quartile for at least two of three years (the high-performance group). The other seven hospitals were assigned to the medium-performance group. Membership in the three groups was kept constant across the three years,

Figure 2-3. *Operating Margins*[a]

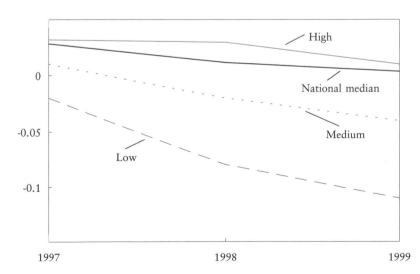

[a]Operating margin values are group means.

Figure 2-4. *Total Margins*[a]

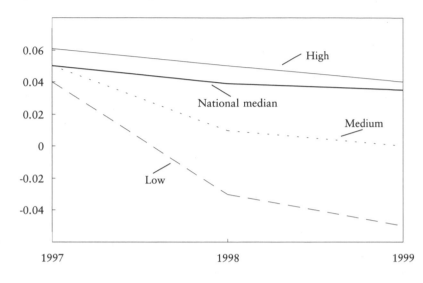

[a]Total margin values are group means.

and the mean results for other financial measures were calculated to provide an understanding of the distribution of values within the AMC sample. Figures 2-3 through 2-8 show key ratios covering the profitability, liquidity, and solvency of the AMCs in the sample (for definitions of the ratios, see table 2-3). Summaries of the performance of the three groups of AMCs follow. They are compared with the national median performance for each ratio, derived from a set of benchmarks produced by the Center for Healthcare Industry Performance Studies (CHIPS).[15] The CHIPS database derives most ratios from a sample of audited financial statements of roughly 1,500 hospitals; their medians for operating profits are derived from Medicare Cost Reports, which are available for nearly all hospitals in the United States.

High-Performance Group

The high-performance group enjoyed positive operating margins throughout the period, although in 1999 the mean operating margin dropped to

15. Center for Healthcare Industry Performance Studies (2000).

Figure 2-5. *Days Cash on Hand, All Sources*[a]

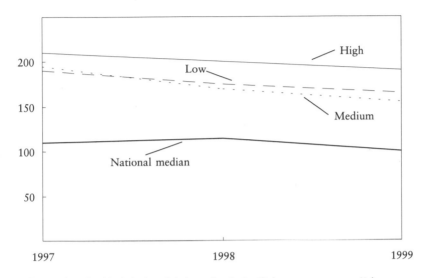

^aDays cash on hand includes board-designated cash classified as noncurrent asset. Values are group means.

roughly 1 percent. In all three years, the high performers outperformed national median trends for operating margins. Operating expenses grew slightly faster than total operating revenues in both 1998 (4 percent and 3 percent respectively) and 1999 (16 percent and 15 percent respectively). Write-downs of nonperforming assets (for example, acquired practices and other acquired businesses) over the period totaled roughly $10 million. Estimated reserves for third-party settlements grew in both years, which may be associated with a conservative statement of net income.[16] Total margins also remained positive but exhibited a steadily declining trend in 1998 and 1999. Again, they remained above the national medians each year, and the decline was driven primarily by the drop in operating margins. Mean days cash on hand from all sources hovered around 200 throughout the period, nearly twice the level of the national median,

16. Estimated third-party reserves represent the amount of revenue that management has determined to set aside (not recognize as revenue) in the event of an adverse third-party settlement in the future. They also represent estimates by management that may be more or less conservatively stated ("conservative" meaning to understate income when in doubt). High/growing reserves may be associated with more conservatively stated net income, and low/shrinking reserves may be associated with less conservatively stated net income.

Figure 2-6. *Equity Financing Ratio*[a]

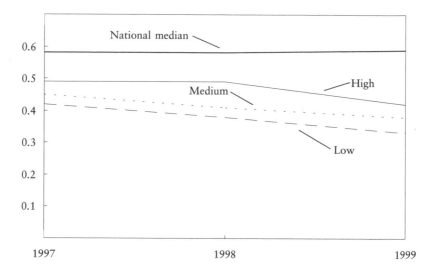

^aValues are group means.

again a favorable financial outcome. Solvency measures (equity financing ratio and cash flow to total debt ratio) show greater debt levels than national medians, representing more financial risk; however, plant age is quite a bit below the national median, indicating greater capital investment in the technologies that give AMCs superior competitive advantages. The reason for the drop in equity financing ratios was substantial increases in long-term debt by two of the four high performers; one borrowed to acquire hospitals, and the other borrowed to build a new campus. Such expansionary investments indicate a confidence about the future that is unlikely to be held by hospitals suffering severe financial distress—or by their creditors. The high-performance group performed better across all measures of financial performance shown here than the other two groups, even though high performance was defined in terms of operating margins only.

Medium-Performance Group

For the 50 percent of the sample representing medium performance, the *trends* across all performance measures resemble those for the low-performance group, but their *values* are higher and less alarming in the

Figure 2-7. *Cash Flow to Total Debt Ratio*[a]

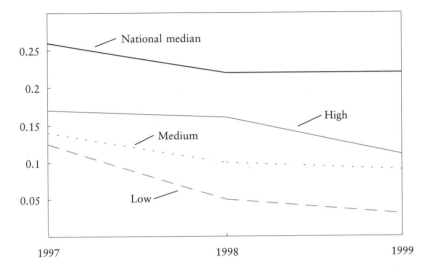

[a]Values are group means.

short run. Several of these hospitals have had to take dramatic steps to stem losses. Operating margins were barely in the black in 1997, but they fell sharply below breakeven in 1998 and again, if a bit less sharply, in 1999. Operating expenses grew faster than total operating revenues in 1998 (means of 9 percent and 6 percent respectively) and in 1999 (5 percent and 3 percent respectively). Write-downs for this group were not large, totaling $15 million over the period for all seven hospitals. However, reserves for third-party liabilities dropped dramatically in 1999 for five of the seven hospitals, with a mean reduction of 27 percent. Total margins, driven by the operating losses, dropped to breakeven in 1999. The number of days of cash on hand also declined, although even in 1999 they were 50 percent above the national median. Equity financing ratios fell from 45 percent to 37 percent, well below the national median. Contributing to the decline in the equity financing ratio was an increase of roughly $250 million in long-term debt (generally seen as a sign of health, as long as it can be repaid) and more than $600 million in transfers of equity out of the reporting entity and into related affiliates. While such transfers clearly weaken the reporting entity's balance sheet, it is not clear whether they went to activities that ultimately may help the AMC financially.

Figure 2-8. *Average Age of Plant*

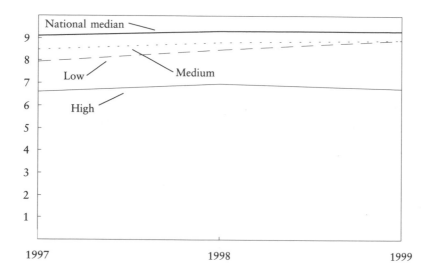

Over the period 1997–99, the leading AMC in terms of transfers was the Hospital of the University of Pennsylvania, which transferred more than $380 million to the medical school, to other hospitals within the system, to faculty practices, and to its primary care network for organizational expenses and acquisitions. Charleston Area Medical Center, which lost a total of $14.7 million on operations, transferred $86 million to affiliates over the same period, which significantly lowered both its equity financing and days-cash-on-hand ratios. Age of plant was greater for this

Table 2-3. *Definitions of Ratios*

Profitability	
Operating margin:	(operating revenue minus expense)/operating revenue
Total margin:	([operating revenue plus investment income] minus expense)/ (operating revenue plus investment income)
Liquidity	
Days cash on hand, all sources:	unrestricted cash and marketable securities, current and noncurrent/([operating expenses minus depreciation]/365)
Solvency	
Equity financing ratio:	unrestricted net assets/total assets
Cash flow to total debt ratio:	(net income plus depreciation)/total debt
Other	
Age of plant:	accumulated depreciation/depreciation expense

group than for both other groups, but it was still below the national median.

Low-Performance Group

The four low-performance hospitals turned in the worst performance of the three groups on most measures. Operating profits in 1997 averaged –4 percent (the level at which the medium group ended up in 1999) and deteriorated, with the biggest decline in 1998. While the other two groups wrote off relatively few nonperforming assets, three of the four hospitals in this group wrote off a total of $172 million over the period, an indication of expensive failed ventures. (Detroit Medical Center led the group, with almost $130 million in write-offs.) Expenses grew much faster than total operating revenues in 1998 (15 percent and 9 percent respectively), with some improvement in 1999 (4 percent and 1 percent respectively), but they were not enough to stop the flow of red ink. Estimated reserves for third parties shrank a mean 10 percent in 1998 and grew by only 1 percent in 1999. Investment income was inadequate to offset operating losses in 1998 or 1999, so total margins sank to –5 percent by 1999.

Days cash on hand dropped from a mean of 196 to 164 over the period, still well above national medians. Solvency measures, however, reached dangerously risky levels, with only a 33 percent equity financing ratio and a 3 percent cash flow to total debt ratio in 1999, putting them well into the bottom quartile for the nation. Plant age trends rose by a full year, from 7.9 to 8.9 years over the period, the fastest aging of the AMC sample (the other two groups aged by roughly .2 years).

Summary

A few AMCs in the middle group experienced pressures throughout the period that were so severe that their financial viability was in doubt. Growth in operating expenses outstripped growth in operating revenues in 1998 and 1999 across all hospital groups, but the divergence was alarming principally for hospitals in the low-performance group. It is likely that one or two in this group will not be able to turn themselves around without massive restructuring, change of ownership, or downsizing. Not all hospitals in the medium-performance group are out of danger either. The Hospital of the University of Pennsylvania, in particular, faced severe operating losses that did not have a major impact on the bottom line until 1999.

Contributing significantly to the financial distress of these hospitals were failed strategies, including mergers and vertical integration efforts.

Most of the AMCs in the sample, however, appeared to be surviving, if not thriving, despite declining operating margins. The pressure on operating margins appears to be systemic, brought on by managed care, Medicaid shortfalls, and Medicare cutbacks, as well as by rising costs for pharmaceuticals, information systems, and new technology. Nevertheless, the management of many AMCs foresaw those revenue pressures and were able to reduce operating costs accordingly. The better-performing AMCs also were able to cut their losses sooner, or they avoided undertaking some of the strategic initiatives that cost others so much.

Conclusions

No single reason accounts for the financial distress or success of AMCs, but an AMC's management capability is a major underlying factor. The low-performance hospitals already were losing money on operations in 1997, so the Balanced Budget Act of 1997 cannot be the primary cause of their problems. High levels of managed care penetration and competition existed in most of the local AMC markets, including those of both high and low performers. The differences among groups in write-offs over the period 1997–1999 suggest that poor business decisions brought on some of the pain experienced by the low performers. Also, expenses grew substantially faster than revenues for the low performers, indicating a serious lack of management control as revenue growth slowed under pressure from payers and competition for patients.

So what should policymakers do about the rising tide of concern over the financial state of AMCs nationwide? Is competition dragging all AMCs down to a state of mediocrity? It does not seem likely.

Policymakers should recognize that the expressions of financial angst are not fully supported by the available facts. Some AMCs indeed are struggling, but most appear to be able to help themselves, especially those with hefty endowments or cash reserves that they were able to generate over the profitable mid-1990s with the aid of tax-exempt debt. (Hospitals chose to borrow for capital needs rather than use internally generated cash, which they invested in marketable securities.) Industrywide data from CHIPS (figure 2-9) show that, while 1998 and 1999 were not great years, the immediately preceding years (1995–97) were the most profitable of the decade. Total margins in 1999 are roughly at the level of total margins

Figure 2-9. *Historical Trends*

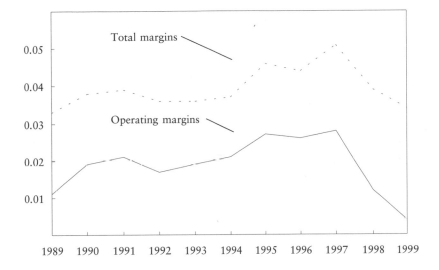

of the early 1990s. Preliminary data suggest that AMC profits are recovering in 2000.[17] Therefore, there does not appear to be an urgent need to do more than already has been done to ensure the viability of most AMCs.

While there may be no need to intervene further to alleviate the financial distress of AMCs, other reforms may be justified for other reasons. Methods of paying for teaching and research could be improved, for example. But those issues should not be resolved in a climate of crisis or in an effort to save failing academic medical centers. In particular, measures that provide unrestricted financial support to AMCs can create unanticipated consequences. Most AMCs exist in competitive markets along with community hospitals. Providing financial support to only one class of competitor gives it advantages that can be used to weaken the others. In Massachusetts, for instance, the financial advantages of AMCs, including indirect medical education payments, strong market appeal, and local political influence, have enabled AMCs to dominate the health care delivery system. Massachusetts patients needing secondary care are far more likely to go to a teaching hospital than are patients in the rest of the country. As a result, the state has unusually high per capita health care costs.[18]

17. Blumenthal (2001).
18. Massachusetts Council of Community Hospitals (2000).

Another reason for caution is that AMCs historically have used their political clout to obtain policy interventions to rescue themselves not only from financial distress but also from the need to change. At the website of the AAMC Forum on the Future of Academic Medicine, a recently published list of the barriers to change in AMCs included the following entries, among others:[19] an entrenched faculty that believes that there is no need for change; top management that is chosen for its nonmanagement skills; the slow pace of decisionmaking and implementation; a sense of entitlement "(Give me dollars and space and leave me alone"); addiction to clinical revenues and current income levels; and the absence of crisis, which can thwart the best efforts of leaders seeking to make necessary changes in strategy or operations.

As one participant in the conference, Bruce Vladeck, noted, "In the 1990s, academic medical centers, along with other hospitals, made hundreds of millions of dollars on inpatient medical-surgical services and squandered them on bad business decisions in physician practices and integration. As a matter of public policy, if we keep increasing the amount we pay hospitals for inpatient care, it is only going to increase the pool of money they have available to lose on their other ventures."

To the extent that AMCs are financially troubled, the problem appears to be a lack of discipline in using the capital that they have rather than a fundamental inadequacy of available resources. Saving one AMC from failure gives other AMCs the green light to maintain their old habits, and it ensures that more failures will mark the future.

COMMENT BY
Ralph Muller

The financial state of academic medicine is receiving considerable attention. It is being discussed not just at this meeting, but also by the Medicare Payment Advisory Commission (MedPAC), the University Health-System Consortium, the Health Care Financing Administration (HCFA), the Association of American Medical Colleges (AAMC), and the American Hospital Association (AHA), among other associations and government agencies.

19. www.aamc.org/about/progemph/forum/barriers.htm

Statistical averages are important, but if we look only at them, we will miss some crucial information. I remember my first statistics course in college, when the professor told the story of the non-swimmer who had waded into a river with an average depth of six inches and drowned. Obviously, some parts of the river were much deeper than average.

I want to address two major kinds of information that one should try to glean from financial reports: Have there been major changes in the financial condition of academic medical centers? And what constitutes financial equilibrium within medical centers?

First, do the financial reports provide any understanding of whether there have been major shifts in financial condition and describe the direction of the turn? In recent years there has been a considerable downturn of overall financial performance among AMCs, especially among the lower quartile of hospitals examined by Nancy Kane. For example, the impact of the Balanced Budget Act (BBA) has placed certain hospitals in deep trouble, and they are finding it difficult to invest in their future renewal. Analysts need to examine why that negative trend is occurring. We know about the price reductions forced by health maintenance organizations and by the BBA cuts. Growth in expenditures is increasing again, after some moderation in the mid to late 1990s. The increase in drug costs is accelerating, a problem that the media have recently noticed. Higher drug costs affect not only Medicare beneficiaries but also hospitals, which have to absorb the higher drug costs within their treatment patterns and fixed payment rates. Public policymakers should be concerned that so much effort is focused on taking care of financially troubled institutions that they neglect general relief for all institutions.

Second, it is important for medical centers and teaching hospitals—as well as other institutions—to be in financial equilibrium, which has at least two characteristics. The first is that growth of expenditures and of revenues are similar—with revenues preferably increasing more than expenses. If I had to pick a most alarming point in Kane's report, it would be that revenue growth is 5 percent below expenditure growth in the lowest quartile of her sample. If that condition persists, it will be disastrous for the affected institutions.

The second characteristic is that the organization has to have sufficient resources to renew its physical and human capital. Most medical centers position themselves in national and local markets as places that are constantly innovating and investing in new people and new technologies. If a medical center cannot renew both its physical facilities and its staff, it cannot remain academically competitive. Financial statements can reveal whether an institution is in equilibrium in both spending and capital renewal.

It is becoming increasingly costly to sustain such equilibrium. In the past, personnel costs constituted the largest cost category; as of 1999, the cost of other inputs, such as drugs, blood products, medical devices, new technologies, and capital renewal, exceeded personnel costs. It is symptomatic of the fact that teaching hospitals are moving toward becoming large intensive care units, spending more and more on such items.

Financial equilibrium also requires that teaching hospitals maintain the real value of their financial reserves. Teaching hospitals occupy a financial position midway between community hospitals—which, by and large, do not have endowments—and universities, which do. Universities have had endowments for many years and tend to have policies for drawing on their endowment—for example, one that stipulates that they may spend as much as 5 percent of the market value of the endowment each year. Hospitals have tended not to use spending rules; instead, they have treated all investment income as available to support operations, even the portion that should be reinvested to maintain the value of financial reserves against inflation. In recent years, superior stock market returns have kept total financial margins of hospitals in the black, while operating margins have been under considerable pressure. Because financial returns dropped sharply starting in early 2000, hospitals that were reporting high total margins as a result of stock market gains from 1995 to 1999 should now show losses.

I urge teaching hospitals to use a university-type spending rule. That is, spend 5 percent of the market value rather than the annual gain. Some already do so. But many have used all of the 15 to 20 percent return on their investments in the last five years to support current operations. When the market offers returns of -10 percent rather than +20 percent, hospitals that have allowed themselves to depend on investment returns to support day-to-day operations will find they lack funds to sustain those operations and support renewal.

A few more points: public policy has a very hard time deciding between worthy and unworthy hospitals. Therefore, over the years, government has tried to use the general reduction of payments from Medicare and Medicaid to bring down all hospitals' payments to see which fall out. The weak financial condition of hospitals in the bottom quartile indicates that while some may recover and survive, others will not. Meanwhile, the policy of reducing payments to all hospitals has consequences for hospitals that perform major health, social, and community roles in the area that they serve.

On average, AMCs in Kane's sample lost $80 million on physician practices and $50 million on insurance products; the combined loss of $130 million is a sizable fraction of their average financial reserves of $250 million. While some of the losses resulted from poorly executed business decisions, many hospitals felt they had to get into or create distributed networks after President Clinton proposed the Health Security Act in 1993. Hospitals suffered major losses as they expanded beyond their core business competency. Investment returns masked those losses for several years, but that situation cannot continue. If portfolios had yielded a normal return of about 10 percent instead of extraordinary 20 percent returns, losses would have been apparent much sooner. In many ways, hospitals shielded themselves from what was happening in their distributed enterprises with investment earnings.

Academic medicine must keep renewing itself to remain a national resource. MedPAC data now indicate that Medicare is paying 104 percent of the cost of care. But private insurance payments have been falling from the 125 to 130 percent of costs that they covered in the early 1990s. Hospital margins have evaporated. Some evidence suggests that some HMOs might be paying more to medical centers that have a geographical hegemony and are therefore able to get better market rates. But overall the margins are insufficient to support renewal. Because medical centers renew themselves through operating earnings, when those earnings dwindle, they cannot invest sufficiently in the future.

The physical and human renewal of medical centers comes out of the margins generated by hospitals. A total margin of 7 to 8 percent—consisting of operating earnings of 3 to 4 percent and investment earnings of 3 to 4 percent—is required to meet the need for capital and program renewal over the long term. The total margin cannot come entirely from investment income because endowments are insufficient and investment returns cannot always be above average. Institutions that have become dependent on large market returns to fund renewal will face considerable difficulties in the next few years.

In summary, Kane has shown that there is a need for revenue and expense equilibrium. It is a disaster to have expenses outpacing revenue by 5 percent. Hospitals in the bottom quartile that are operating at a loss of 8 percent are starting to fail. She also has shown that hospitals must use investment income responsibly. The sampled hospitals have an average of

$250 million of investments. But they must be prudent about how they use the income and not depend on supernormal returns. Next she has shown that medical centers must have disciplined ways to renew themselves in the future. They compete in national markets for students, faculty, and research grants. Many are in trouble, but even troubled organizations, such as CareGroup, must compete in the market for new people.

Institutions must continue to try to renew themselves and to stay competitive nationally and locally. The question is how they are going to obtain the necessary resources. The stock market will not perform as it did from 1995 to 2000. Philanthropy also depends on a robust stock market. The key to long-run success is a strong and balanced flow of income—from operations (including public support), investments, and philanthropy.

COMMENT BY
James Reuter

I was surprised and pleased to see that Nancy Kane's excellent analysis was not based on some version of either the annual survey of the American Hospital Association (AHA) or Medicare cost data. It is refreshing to see a serious attempt to seek alternative sources of data to address fundamental and significant questions about the current financial status of academic medical centers.

The use of new sources, however, creates a significant challenge for the researcher, particularly if the results are intended to contribute to public policy debates; while more commonly used data have their limitations, they are useful for communicating with policymakers. Researchers may debate the true significance of Medicare margins or the levels of uncompensated care reported on AHA surveys, but to policymakers, those constructions are old and trusted friends. Policymakers know what it means—at least politically—when Medicare margins turn up or down. So a researcher who uses a new source must accept the challenge of working through a careful presentation of all of the definitions and interpretations of the new data source and measures. Kane's data appear to allow a mix of reporting units, with particular emphasis on the clinical mission. Sometimes data are based solely on the operations of an AMC's hospital; in other cases, the data also include the operations of the medical school or faculty practice plan.

Over the last several years, I have been working with the Commonwealth Task Force on Academic Health Centers, which has tried to put data from the various elements of AMCs together in a way that makes sense and allows consideration of the AMC as a whole. Combining existing data sources has several disadvantages for accomplishing that goal. In particular, one must deal with the problem of double-counting the cross-subsidies. Revenues to one unit of an AMC (and resulting expenses) may be reported also as an expense to another. Both the Association of American Medical Colleges and the University HealthSystem Consortium have engaged in efforts to develop data that would describe the flow of funds within AMCs.

My understanding of Kane's data is that some of the reporting units represent complete AMCs while others represent just the clinical enterprises. While the data presented are based on a sample of convenience, it should be possible to design a sample of reporting institutions that would reflect the complete operations of some subset of AMCs. I would encourage the author to pursue a more informative sample in subsequent work.

We keep getting separate pieces of information on each component of AMCs but those pieces often do not really talk to each other. Nonetheless, I think that trying to put those data together in a larger context is important because the result will shed light on AMCs underlying financial strength.

A key aspect of the financial health of AMCs is their ability to survive economic downturns. Like every other organization, AMCs experience economic cycles; the question is whether they have the assets to carry them through. Kane's analysis provides important new insights on that question. Some institutions are much more fragile than others. The margin—the ratio of cash flow to total debt and debt service—clearly suggests that when things go bad, the financial health of some AMCs can deteriorate very quickly. My own institution, Georgetown University, provides a ready example. In the early 1990s, Georgetown was in an expansive mode. It used cash flow from clinical operations to support investments in research. In a very short period, things deteriorated so much that the board of trustees felt obliged to divest the university of the clinical enterprise to protect its overall financial status.

These results suggest that it may be fruitful to apply the same or similar measures to all AMCs to an effort to identify institutions at risk. Public policy initiatives and support could then target problems much more effectively. At the same time, institutions at risk could develop plans or curtail expansions in order to improve their ability to survive short-term adverse operating results.

Another important aspect of Kane's presentation is the documentation of the increasing complexity of AMCs and their financial relationships. In some cases, hundreds of millions of dollars were being lost, gained, and otherwise transferred. I do not believe that any of those financial relationships and dependencies would have been revealed through traditional financial surveys and cost reports; nevertheless, those relationships obviously have major implications for the financial health of the AMCs involved. New analyses and sources of data are necessary to reveal the "true" financial health of AMCs. Kane suggests some, and researchers should seek others.

Kane's presentation also documents the need for AMCs to maintain high cash and investment balances if they are to remain financially healthy. In an era of declining surpluses from clinical missions and enterprises, AMCs need to identify new sources of regular income to subsidize their academic and research missions. One obvious approach, which AMCs increasingly are using, is to build up their investment and endowment portfolios. The run-up in the stock market inflated the returns for many institutions, and one hopes that AMCs have not planned on the unrealistic assumption that they can be sustained indefinitely. Nevertheless, Kane clearly suggests that those funds fill in part of the gap reflected in declining margins and help AMCs hold their own. Endowment earnings and annual giving have obvious and significant benefits for institutions. Many AMCs are aggressively building their development campaigns to fill gaps in traditional sources of support.

I interpret Kane's presentation to reconfirm the need for AMCs to exercise caution when investing in new opportunities—whether in their clinical, research, or educational missions. Many investments, such as those that many AMCs made in physician practices or community hospitals, may take years to show a positive return, if ever. As illustrated by the experience of Georgetown and other institutions, financial losses can build very rapidly. In my view, AMCs' first responsibility is to secure the financial future of their core activities.

COMMENT BY
Peter Van Etten

I have to begin with a disclaimer: I have been out of the academic medical center (AMC) mainstream for a year. The industry changes fast, so my perspective may be somewhat dated, but I doubt that there have been fundamental changes in the last year that would change my comments.

The financial status of AMCs has been debated for many years. On one hand, MedPAC and various studies published in *Health Affairs* have concluded that there is little evidence of deteriorating profitability, in particular as a result of recent changes to the Medicare program. On the other hand, the Association of American Medical Colleges has provided compelling evidence of deteriorating margins and several major AMCs have reported significant losses in the last few years.

I find it distressing that this debate has been going on for all of the twenty-five years I have been involved in academic medicine. A large part of the problem is that the only easily comparable information on AMCs is the audited financial reports of their hospitals, which show only one aspect of AMCs. They omit practice plans, as well as research and educational programs. A vast web of cross-subsidies exists in most AMCs among clinical care, research, and teaching programs, as well as among AMCs' various institutional elements. AMCs' profitability will never be adequately measured without a better understanding of the activities of all their components.

I agree with James Robinson that Nancy Kane's analysis is well designed. The fifteen AMCs in the sample are a reasonably good cross-section, except that no West Coast institutions are represented. I think that Kane did a good job of dealing with the lack of consistency in the published financial reports. Her analysis provides clear evidence of declining margins at those institutions; what is not clear is the reason for the decline. She suggests two reasons. One is that contractual allowances are rising at a faster rate than gross patient service revenues. That could be due to declining activity or greater discounts. The second reason is that costs are rising faster than revenue. It is interesting that the study does not show that declining profitability is the result of increasing bad debt.

One of the most important findings is that the AMCs in the top quartile are doing reasonably well while those in the bottom quartile are getting much poorer. That variation has not been examined by others, who have looked at means and medians in performing profitability analyses of AMCs. From personal experience, I would suggest that hospitals experiencing declining profitability often find that their losses accelerate, because expense reductions designed to improve profitability often result in revenue declines, exacerbating financial distress.

So what could be done to improve the analysis? The addition of West Coast institutions would provide a more complete picture. AMCs in California are in a particularly precarious situation. The significant subsidies provided by the University of California to its AMCs tend to obscure that problem, which results in large part from two sources: the large discounts that private payers have secured, often far greater than in other parts of the country, and the fact that California's Medicaid payments are among the lowest in the country.

While an understanding of the profitability of all elements of AMCs, not just their hospitals, would improve the analysis, few institutions have determined the profitability of their various components. Most for-profit organizations are managed with extensive information regarding profitability by business segment; however, that is not the case with AMCs. What is needed is a uniform approach to what sometimes is called funds-flow analysis; that requires understanding the cross-subsidies that are a fundamental aspect of most AMCs. Often there is political risk in performing such analyses because recipients of subsidies fear that they will lose their subsidies if it is widely known that they receive them. It is particularly critical to understand how the funds flow within an AMC affects faculty behavior. The University HealthSystem Consortium and Ernst and Young designed an effective approach to analyzing funds flow that has been used in a limited number of AMCs. The analysis also would be improved by providing a better understanding of the differences between the top and bottom quartiles.

General Discussion

Bruce Vladeck wondered whether industrywide acceptance of a false premise—that inpatient medical and surgical services is a dying industry—is the reason little progress has been made in the past twenty-five years in understanding whether academic medical centers are profitable. According to that notion, institutions must diversify in order to survive. Vladeck noted that in the 1990s many hospitals, including AMCs, made hundreds of millions of dollars on inpatient medical and surgical services but squandered the profits by making bad business decisions in other ventures, such as running physician practices and provider-owned health insurance plans. Most recent efforts to find solutions to the financial problems of AMCs have focused on Medicare revenues and indirect medical education, perhaps because the data are highly visible and the regulations themselves are most susceptible to the political process. Vladeck suggested that that focus is misplaced, because he suspects that costly and unprofitable faculty practice plans are at the root of the financial crisis.

Vladeck also pointed out that while Ralph Muller claimed that total operating margins of 7 to 8 percent were necessary to sustain academic health centers, the historical average is only about half of that. He argued that there is risk involved in looking at a very short historical period and generalizing from that. Because of accelerating technological change and the increasing role of drug companies, however, margins necessary for renewal could be significantly greater in the future than they were in the past.

Spencer Foreman agreed with Vladeck that faculty practices are a major problem, citing his own institution's yearly $60 million dollar subsidy to an unprofitable faculty practice. He stressed that although abandoning faculty practices is difficult, their losses must be curbed. He suggested that most faculty at AMCs may live in a cultural bubble, mistakenly thinking that they do not have to adapt to change.

Foreman noted that excess capacity causes some facilities to offer services below average (but above marginal) cost. He also noted that the most troubled institutions often are safety-net providers; somebody typically comes in to bail them out, perpetuating the excess capacity problem.

Herbert Pardes said that hospitals face both current revenue/cost pressure and difficulty attracting capital; the strong stock market obscured the problem, but a declining market has made it more visible. Kenneth Shine stressed the high cost of new technologies; in addition, drug prices are increasing at an annual rate of about 14 to 17 percent. Shine pointed out that AMCs, which invent the technologies, are largely responsible for those trends, which in turn cause the AMCs major financial problems. The more innovative academic medical centers are, the more financial pressure they face. He cautioned that AMCs must look carefully at when and how they use their innovations.

Pardes suggested that decisions on the introduction of technology should not be the responsibility of the academic medical center alone. The government, or the country as a whole, has decided to make a massive investment in medical research. The mandate to develop new and better ways to identify, prevent, and treat disease is something that AMCs can respond to, but they cannot make the ultimate decision on how to use a new technology in isolation from society as a whole.

Robert Reischauer asked Nancy Kane to clarify whether the various quartiles consisted of hospitals whose position was fixed by their rank in 1997 or whether the membership of those quartiles and the number of hospitals varied over time. If the latter, he observed that it would be difficult to know what to make of the trends. He also wished to see an examination by quartile of occupancy rates for inpatient and volume of outpatient services over time. Kane replied that hospitals did not stay in their initial quartile over the three years but that the number of hospitals remained the same.

Lawrence Lewin commended Kane's effort, but agreed with James Reuter that a complete analysis of the financial state of academic medical centers would require data on the rest of the enterprise. Those data are not readily available, however, and they would be hard to analyze if they were because even though the missions of AMCs differ, they are interrelated, making it difficult to assign costs to particular missions. Clinical care, for example, is intertwined with education and research.

Al Dobson noted that in New York, Connecticut, Pennsylvania, and Massachusetts legislatures seem to believe that medical centers are doing far better than they claim, that they are hiding money, and that they actually are quite rich. Dobson said that in a study of financially distressed hospitals in Connecticut he found, as Kane reported, that the inpatient services were profitable and were cross-subsidizing operations that posted losses. He wondered which hospitals would be hit by the decline in stock prices during the second half of 2000. He asked whether Kane had information on whether hospitals invest mostly in bonds or in stocks.

Dobson reported that his research in Connecticut found that in about one-fourth of hospitals, everything seemed to be falling apart at once and fast—occupancy was down, competition was tough, and there was a cost/revenue squeeze. As they began to draw down their endowments, they quickly became insolvent and frequently defaulted.

Dobson pointed out that a major problem is that no one is paying cost. In Massachusetts, commercial payments cover only 95 to 98 percent of costs, Medicaid payments are down at 77 percent, and Medicare payments are a bit less than breakeven. Commercial insurers pay roughly 105 percent in Pennsylvania and 119 percent overall. If most payers pay less than cost, Dobson noted, one is in a very difficult business.

Shine argued that hospitals are not very good at running ambulatory facilities or physician practices. He pointed out that one of the reasons that inpatient financial operations look so strong is that inpatient costs sometimes are assigned to outpatient services. Moreover, the faculty often does not have a vested interest in the operations of the hospital. He asked whether not only practice plans, but also all ambulatory operations, should be spun off so that incentives for accurate reporting would improve. Without accurate reporting it is hard to have sound management decisions.

Brian Biles commented that academic medical centers have been claiming financial distress for twenty-five years but that their allegations have yet to be convincingly demonstrated. He asked Kane whether the institutions in the bottom quartile are now actually hitting a wall—that is, barring a national response, whether those institutions will be forced to shut down within the next five or ten years.

Robert Dickler mentioned that it is important to remember that there always will be a bottom 25 percent. He also wanted to make explicit that, unlike "hospital" and "medical school," "AMC" has no agreed-upon legal or financial definition; consequently, these terms should be used with care. For example, money occasionally may move among the various components of an AMC, but funds usually are aligned with each component. And while everyone wants to share the profits of other units, no one wants to assume any of the losses.

Henry Aaron asked whether it was a good or a bad thing to have the bottom quartile falling apart. Reuter replied that health plans want to keep weak hospitals open while strong hospitals want to close them. Public policy also is divided. Antitrust groups want to keep excess capacity to stimulate competition, whereas payers, such as HCFA, want to end it because it raises costs. Competition is good; excess costs are not. Pardes was of the opinion that closing hospitals in the bottom quartile could be worth considering. The danger in sustaining excess capacity, he argued, is that it weakens all hospitals, threatening to debase the quality of the modest number of top-quality hospitals.

Reischauer stressed the importance of distinguishing between levels and rates of growth. Higher levels of spending by AMCs may be necessary to sustain some institutions as leaders, but sustained higher rates of growth could lead to an undesirable gap in quality between academic health centers and other hospitals.

Nancy Kane responded that academic medical centers compete not only with each other but also with other hospitals and other providers; providing advantages to academic medical centers can destroy their competitors. In Massachusetts, for example, AMCs have used their financial and market strength to drive community hospitals out of business. She acknowledged uncertainty about whether her sample was representative. She said that by selling assets and restructuring, some faltering medical centers probably would recover, even without help from the government, but that some may be in a downward spiral from which they cannot escape. She estimated that as much as 65 percent of medical center unrestricted investment portfolios are invested in equities. Kane disputed the notion that those institutions should not spend more than about 5 to 6 percent of the market value of their unrestricted investment portfolios each year. Using some of the profits from the 1990s probably will be necessary to compensate for loses from poor strategic decisions made previously.

Kane agreed that understanding the relationships among the components of AMCs is critical to analyzing their problems; however, those relationships are not reported in any standard way. All data are self-reported; they are not subject to audit, and they may not be reliable. For that reason, case studies are the only plausible way to get at the heart of some of the issues that have been raised.

She also pointed out that faculty practices and owned practices of community doctors are problematic. Owning community doctors is the source of the biggest losses and most troubling problems. Academic health centers have been wrestling with faculty practice plans for a long time, but they have formed business relationships with community doctors only recently. Study of faculty practice plans is hampered by the fact that each department has its own way of setting things up.

Kane closed by expressing weariness with the public perception that academic medical centers are suffering great losses and that therefore policymakers must do something to save them. AMCs, she said, are the most powerful units in the health care system. Congress listens to them, and they receive breaks that many other health care institutions do not. They are much better organized than any other group of providers. She believes that the real problem is AMCs' lack of discipline in applying and using the capital that they have rather than any inability to make new investments.

References

American Hospital Association. 1990. *Comparative Analysis of Annual Survey and Medicare Cost Report Margin Data.* Technical Report E-90-08. Submitted to the Prospective Payment Assessment Commission. Chicago.

American Institute of Certified Public Accountants. 1998. *AICPA Audit and Accounting Guide for Health Care Organizations.* New York.

Arrick, Martin, Kenneth Rodgers, and Sharon Gigante. 2000. *Special Report: Health Care at a Crossroads.* Standard & Poor's Credit Week Municipal Report (October 23).

Blumenthal, David. 2001. "Unhealthy Hospitals: Addressing the Trauma in Academic Medicine." *Harvard Magazine* (March-April): 29–31.

Blumenthal, David, and Samuel O. Thier. 1998. "Leveling the Playing Field: A Report of the Commonwealth Fund Task Force on Academic Health Centers." *Journal of Urban Health: Bulletin of the New York Academy of Medicine* 75(2): 300–46.

Burns, Lawton R., John Cacciamani, James Clement, and Welman Aquino. 2000. "The Fall of the House of AHERG: The Allegheny Bankruptcy." *Health Affairs* (January/February): 7– 41.

Casey, Michael. 1999. "Penn's Losses: An Omen for Teaching Facilities?" *Medical Industry Today* (November 9).

Center for Healthcare Industry Performance Studies. 2000. *2001 Almanac of Hospital Financial and Operating Indicators: A Comprehensive Benchmark of the Nation's Hospitals.* Ingenix Publishing Group.

Gaynor, Pamela. 2000. "Investing a Lot in Medicine." *Pittsburgh Post-Gazette.* Business News. (July 2).

Healthcare Financial Management Association. 1994. *Principles and Practices Board Statement Number 18: Public Disclosure of Financial and Operating Information by Healthcare Providers.*

Herbert, Bob. 1999. "Hospitals in Crisis." *New York Times* (April 15): Section A, 31.

Kane, Nancy M., and Stephen Magnus. 2001. "The Medicare Cost Report and the Limits of Hospital Accountability: Improving Financial Accounting Data." *Journal of Health Policy, Politics, and Law* 26 (1): 83–107.

Knox, Richard, and Aaron Zitner. 1999. "Who Will Pay? Teaching Hospitals Struggle with Costs; Condition: Critical." *Boston Globe* (June 27): p. A1.

Marquis, Julie. 2000. "Many Academic Medical Centers Struggling Financially, Panel Says." *Los Angeles Times* (May 5): A 28.

Massachusetts Council of Community Hospitals. 2000. *A Study of the Condition of Massachusetts Community Hospitals and Prospects for the Future.* Peabody, Mass.

Powers, Scott. 2000. "Searching for a Cure, OSU Hospitals among Teaching Institutions Facing Financial Pinch." *Columbus Dispatch* (February 20): 1G.

Rodgers, Kenneth W. , Lisa Zuckerman, and Terry Goode. 2000. *An Overview of Academic Medical Centers.* Standard & Poor's Public Finance Report (November 30).

CHAPTER THREE

Academic Medical Centers and the Economics of Innovation in Health Care

James C. Robinson

Academic medical centers are caught in a backlash between the conventional wisdom of yesteryear, when bigger was regarded as better, and the conventional wisdom of today, which holds that AMCs should downsize and divest themselves of affiliated community hospitals, long-term and home health care services, primary care practices, and other ancillary programs. This chapter examines the efficient boundaries of the academic medical center through the lens of the economic literature on technological innovation and organizational integration.

To appropriate the economic benefits of innovation in the absence of intellectual property protections, organizations need to combine innovations with complementary assets such as production facilities, distribution channels, inventory of specialized components, and marketing mechanisms. If they do not, they will not be able to set prices sufficient to cover the cost of research and development, and the benefits of innovation will accrue primarily to suppliers, distributors, and competitors. Similar principles apply to the efforts of AMCs to create sustainable financing for their four key pursuits: laboratory research on the etiology of diseases; biotechnology; clinical trials; and the provision of specialty services. Academic institutions can choose to own the activities and assets necessary to ensure their ability to appropriate the economic benefits of their innovations, or they can enter into contracts or partnerships with independent organizations.

Academic medical centers today face unprecedented challenges to their financial stability and organizational mission. Long the undisputed pinnacle of the health care hierarchy, many university hospitals now find it difficult to differentiate themselves from community institutions, freestanding ambulatory diagnostic and surgical facilities, independent physician networks, contract research organizations, and a host of less costly competitors. The current difficulties of AMCs are ironic in light of their historic dedication to the pursuit of innovation in science, technology, and service provision, which is central to the "new economy." Despite those difficulties, AMCs have the potential to dominate the market for the newest and best in clinical care if they can find ways to appropriate the economic benefits of their activities for themselves rather than watch those benefits dissipate among their competitors.

As demonstrated repeatedly in other high-technology sectors, successful appropriation of the benefits of innovation requires the alignment of organizational and research strategies. Yet many medical centers devoted the past decade to building clinical conglomerates under the mistaken impression that economies of scale and scope would accrue to those entities that brought the entire continuum of care under one organizational umbrella rather than to those that selectively acquired assets to leverage their activities. Many AMCs are devoting the current decade to the pursuit of market monopoly and political power; few appear to be monitoring the strategies and structures of other knowledge-based organizations that depend on innovation for their success and failure, including those in biotechnology, pharmaceuticals, and medical devices and in the non–health-related information economy.

This chapter examines the prospects of academic medical centers in light of the economic theory of innovation. AMCs undertake many activities in addition to research, development, and the diffusion of knowledge, and they serve many masters; in particular, they also provide medical education, offer specialized services, and treat the indigent. Focusing on research does seem valid, however, because scientific inquiry is what distinguishes academic medical centers from otherwise similar hospital systems. I first explain the economic theory of innovation, emphasizing the importance of devising mechanisms to capture the financial returns on research and development activites if the innovating organization is to be self-sustaining. I then consider the potential for economic appropriation of the benefits of research in the four key areas mentioned previously. I try to maintain a balanced view of the advantages and disadvantages of large organizations. I do not believe that there is a sound basis for either yesterday's belief that bigger is better or today's belief that academic medical centers should sell off, shut down, and outsource everything. No one can confidently foretell the future of the academic medical center, but it certainly does not lie in emulating the Cheshire cat, which "downsized" beginning with the tail and ended with naught but the smile.

The Appropriation of Innovation

The ability to appropriate the economic benefits of innovation is the key to sustaining research and development activities in any sector.[1] The marketplace is littered with the corpses of once-prominent firms that were unable to embed their innovations in products and services that could be sold at a price sufficient to cover research costs; in the absence of successful appropriation strategies, a company loses the economic benefits of its innovations to competitors, suppliers, distributors, or customers.[2] Descriptions follow of four methods that exist in the contemporary economy for appropriating the economic benefits of research and development.

Research grants

Government, industry, and philanthropic entities often make grants to fund some forms of research without demanding ownership or special control; such grants can obviate the need for the research organization to embed its innovations in a salable product or service. But there is significant competition among organizations for research support. Most AMCs find themselves beset by ever-increasing numbers and types of competitors for government support, including nearby medical centers, nonmedical university departments, and large community hospitals, and for industry research support, including in-house research departments at pharmaceutical and biotechnology firms, medical device manufacturers, and contract research organizations.

Intellectual property protection

Patents, trademarks, copyrights, and other forms of intellectual property rights afford innovators an exclusive, although temporary, right to use or to license others to use the products of their research activities. However,

1. Dosi (1988); Nelson (1990); Pavitt (1984).
2. Teece (1992, 1998).

intellectual property rights are effective only in sectors in which the innovation can be clearly described and distinguished from imitations, as in the chemical, pharmaceutical, and biotechnology industries. Moreover, patent restrictions are subject to evasion through development of similar, though not identical, products; that threat leads innovators in some industries to rely more on trade secrets than on patents (for example, the formula for Coca-Cola). The use of patent protection to extract the full economic value of health-related innovations is socially controversial, however, as is evident in the contemporary demonization of the research-intensive pharmaceutical industry. The pyramiding of patent protections in the information technology, genomic, and biotechnology sectors is alleged to lead to social underinvestment in follow-on research and development activity, and the contemporary policy debate may lead to a weakening of intellectual property protections.[3]

Monopoly Power

To the extent that a firm is the sole provider of a particular product or service in a market, it can set prices to recuperate the costs of research and development.[4] For example, its government-guaranteed monopoly enabled ATT to finance extensive research in telecommunications technology for most of the twentieth century. After the government breakup of the firm on antitrust grounds, it became necessary to find new sources of research support. Monopoly power may favor research by allowing a company not only to raise revenues but also to standardize systems and ensure the compatibility of components. It has been argued that compatibility benefits justify monopoly or quasi-monopoly structures in sectors with rapidly evolving technologies.[5] In general, however, the world economy is becoming more, rather than less, competitive due to globalization, deregulation, privatization, and the rapid reduction of transportation and communication costs.

Complementary Assets

Without grants, strong patent protection, or monopoly power, companies investing in research and development activities must embed their innova-

---

3. Heller and Eisenberg (1998).
4. Schumpeter (1962); Cohen and Levin (1989).
5. Shapiro and Varian (1999).

tions in products and services that sell for more than marginal cost. To do so, innovators must own or control complementary assets such as manufacturing facilities, brand names, sales and distribution channels, key raw and processed materials, or the important inputs and components in the supply chain.[6] Without control of strategic assets, innovators will be unable to prevent competing companies from imitating their innovations.

Much of the research performed by academic medical centers traditionally has been supported by government grants and hence falls under the first form of appropriating the economic benefits of innovation. As has become evident in recent years, however, government grants often do not cover the full costs of bench and, especially, of clinical research. As a result, AMCs must cross-subsidize grant-financed research with profits from other services; however, declines in clinical revenues resulting from government cutbacks and managed care contracting are eroding those cross-subsidies. Academic medical centers have sought to appropriate the benefits of some innovations, especially those related to biotechnology, through aggressive pursuit and enforcement of patents. That technique also is limited by competition from freestanding biotechnology firms, pharmaceutical giants, and contract research organizations eager to garner the same economic benefits.[7]

In short, AMCs increasingly find themselves in the same position as research-intensive firms in other sectors, where competition grows fiercer every year. Grants often do not cover full research costs, yet competition for them steadily intensifies. Patents can be used to protect only a limited range of innovations for a limited period of time; yet there is a competitive race to obtain them too. Monopoly power is a chimera in most of the metropolitan areas where teaching hospitals are concentrated.

Academic medical centers therefore must focus on the fourth appropriation strategy, that of acquiring or contracting for the complementary assets that permit them to command above-average prices for innovative services even in competitive markets. It is in light of that imperative that the efforts of AMCs over the past decade to acquire community hospitals, primary care practices, subacute care facilities, ambulatory surgery centers, and insurance entities needs to be evaluated.

6. Teece (1986); Cohen and Zysman (1987).
7. Rettig (2000).

Organizational Boundaries

Innovative organizations that lack monopoly power and strong intellectual property protections must rely on organizational structure to appropriate the economic benefits of their research activities. Successful commercialization in competitive markets typically requires that new knowledge or innovations be combined with other assets or capabilities. To the extent that those ancillary capabilities are generic and available at competitive prices, innovators need not bring them in house through merger or acquisition; if, however, they are specialized or otherwise not available in the marketplace, the innovator must build internal capabilities and develop meaningful partnerships with selected outside suppliers or risk losing the benefits of its research investment to imitators. The boundaries of the organization, defined in terms of which capabilities are owned and which are obtained through contract, must be evaluated in terms of the relative advantages of internal and external coordination.

Advantages and Disadvantages of Integration

Organizations are best interpreted as mechanisms of governance designed to bring together diverse individuals, units, and divisions for joint purposes without having to incur the costs of searching and contracting for services or goods in the market. The leaders in an integrated organization have the authority to establish new priorities, monitor the flow of information, create new incentives, and redirect individuals and assets from one project to another. The modern pharmaceutical corporation exemplifies the potential of an integrated organization. It sponsors basic and applied research; develops and tests products; and manufactures, distributes, and markets products to physicians and patients, all primarily with internally owned and employed assets.

It is important to recognize that fully integrated companies are rare in the non–health-related economy, a fact that constitutes implicit evidence of the disadvantages of internal ownership and coordination. For example, even the largest and wealthiest pharmaceutical firms often find it advantageous to contract with, cooperate with, or invest in independent biotechnology firms rather than bring biotechnology research and development activities in house. The disadvantages of integration include the generic liabilities that attend all large and complex organizations, but also more specific liabilities that vary from one asset and function to another.

First, capital requirements may be prohibitive. Investors and creditors become increasingly wary—and demand increasingly steep risk premiums—as debt burdens grow and shareholder equity is diluted. Second, scale economies may be sacrificed. An independent supplier or distributor that contracts with multiple innovators may be able to achieve lower costs and better quality through the volume and experience gained from multiple relationships. Those advantages would not be available were every innovator to build its own (necessarily smaller) supply or distribution division. Third, integrated companies may not be able to keep up with technological change in all sectors. Products and services that involve rapidly changing technologies require the producer to keep up with the latest developments in multiple sectors, an overwhelming task. Outsourcing allows a firm with leading-edge technology in one component to access the best technology in other components without having to lead change in those sectors. Fourth, integrated companies may lose contact with changing customer needs. Nonexclusive contracting with outside suppliers indirectly brings a business into contact with a wide range of end-users who purchase from competitors. Demand changes rapidly in technologically dynamic industries, and outside contractors can offer invaluable information on trends in product features, prices, and performance.

Access to complementary assets and capabilities can be obtained through ownership, contracting, or a multitude of hybrid mechanisms that combine elements of ownership and contracting, including partial cross-ownership, reciprocal selling, exclusive purchase agreements, multiyear contracts, technology swaps, patent pooling, joint research ventures, and joint marketing initiatives. The most dynamic sectors of the contemporary economy, including telecommunications, computer hardware and software, Internet services, and biotechnology, are characterized by the multiplicity and complexity of their relationships with independent suppliers, distributors, and even competitors.[8]

The Old Conventional Wisdom and the New

Only yesterday the conventional wisdom in the health care industry held that academic medical centers should expand the range of their services, merge with or acquire erstwhile competitors, and form integrated delivery systems. Today's conventional wisdom maintains that AMCs must pur-

8. Pisano (1991); Powell (1987).

sue precisely the opposite organizational strategy. The bankruptcy of the Allegheny system in Philadelphia, perhaps the epitome of medical empire building, caused a reversal in consultants' advice and managerial sentiment. The well-publicized difficulties of University of California (San Francisco)/Stanford, Penn State/Geisinger, University of Pennsylvania, CareGroup, and others swelled the rising tide of scorn heaped on integrated delivery systems. Moody's has ascribed its downgrade of hospitals' and AMCs' bond ratings largely to efforts at vertical and horizontal integration,[9] and Standard & Poor's, among numerous others, has observed that nonprofit hospitals cannot continue to rely on investment profits to cover operating losses.[10]

The investor-owned hospital chains have emerged from financial and judicial purgatory with a renewed appetite for helping academic medical centers take money-losing assets off their balance sheets.[11] Consultants and turnaround specialists now swarm over AMCs, advising divestment of primary care physician practices, closure of provider-sponsored HMOs, spin-off of community affiliates, sale or shutdown of ancillary facilities, and reconsideration of the notion that the university hospital should be the flagship of some clinical armada.[12]

The sober sentiment of the moment is well-founded in the economic theory of organization and in the bitter experiences of integrated health care. Focus, transparency, accountability, provision of incentives, and speedy response time are virtues that AMCs need to nurture. Yet the facile turnaround from yesterday's conventional wisdom to today's threatens to produce an overreaction that forces short-term write-offs and limits the long-term ability of the academic medical center to pursue its four-part mission of research, teaching, patient care, and safety net. The research mission, in particular, has important implications for the scale and scope of an AMC, and insight into establishing organizational boundaries can be derived by considering the boundaries of other knowledge-based enterprises.

9. Goldstein and others (2000).

10. Zuckerman, Rodgers, and Goode (2000, www.standardandpoors.com/ratingsdirect [November 30]).

11. Feinstein and Raskin (2000).

12. Hunter (2000).

Appropriation of Innovation in Medicine

The economic literature on innovation and appropriation focuses on the high-technology manufacturing sector; it does not deal explicitly with the innovative activities of the academic medical center. Yet many of the basic principles are applicable to medical centers as they struggle to finance their research mission through the sale of products and services that flow from bench and clinical research activities. A major portion of academic medical center research will continue to be funded by extramural grants that require free dissemination of the findings to all interested parties. But the incessant discussion in AMCs over how to translate research into patents, obtain higher prices for higher-quality care, retain industry support for clinical trials, and manage joint ventures with outside firms or their own entrepreneurial physicians underscores the importance of economic appropriation to AMCs' survival. The appropriation strategy itself and the roles therein for ownership, contracts, and partnerships will vary across different forms of laboratory and clinical research. Preliminary insights can be obtained by taking a brief look at the four principal forms of research performed in the academic medical center today.

Laboratory Research Excluding Biotechnology

With the exception of biotechnology and some innovations relevant to medical devices, much of the laboratory research conducted in AMCs must be supported through extramural grants rather than salable products.[13] The National Institutes of Health and other government agencies always will be the major underwriters of scientific research; that fact does not imply, however, that organizational boundaries and questions of whether to build internal capabilities or to contract or partner with other organizations to obtain them are irrelevant. In order to compete effectively for extramural support, AMCs must maintain an efficient organizational boundary, not burden themselves with overhead from inessential and not fully self-supporting activities.[14] Much of the contemporary hand-wringing concerning overinvestment in community facilities, provider-sponsored HMOs, and primary care practices has centered on the shortfall between operating rev-

---

13. Commonwealth Fund (1999).
14. Griner and Blumenthal (1998); Blumenthal, Weissman, and Griner (1999).

enues and operating costs. Over the longer term, however, the most significant liability of expansion plans may prove to be diversion of effort and accretion of administrative overhead, which hinder AMCs in competing for research support. In the space of a decade many clinical services have deteriorated from being profitable activities that could subsidize underfunded research programs to being unprofitable activities that distract the institution from its research mission. In that context, academic medical centers desperately need better internal cost accounting mechanisms that allow them to understand the full costs of research and nonresearch activities and thereby identify the size of implicit cross-subsidies.

Biotechnology and Medical Devices

Bench research with profitable applications in biotechnology, pharmaceuticals, and medical devices clearly raises a different set of issues, as the economic appropriation of innovation in the conventional sense is possible. Universities—after watching with dismay the appropriation of university-sponsored research by independent companies, many launched by former faculty members—now have gone far down the path of pursuing patents, licenses, partnerships, and ownership in private firms.[15] In most instances, AMCs do not move all the way into manufacturing, distribution, marketing, and sales but contract and partner with independent organizations. But the range of strategic options remains wide. At one end of the spectrum, an AMC can patent its discoveries and license their use to other parties. Better returns on investments often can be obtained, however, if the university remains involved in how its patented discoveries are used by combining them with other patents and with nonpatented processes. That form of continued involvement typically requires an ownership position in the outside firm. It is a truism in the technology sector that most economic rewards are obtained through growth in the value of the enterprise, measured in stock price appreciation, rather than through revenues from any one particular product or service. Needless to say, it is imperative for AMCs to develop a careful policy for industrial investments and partnerships to avoid undermining their larger social role.[16]

15. Kenney (1986).
16. Martin and Kasper (2000).

Clinical Trials

The market for clinical trials is becoming more competitive as second-tier medical centers solicit the same pharmaceutical company and government support formerly monopolized by universities and as nonacademic contract research organizations bring together community facilities and physicians into lower-cost networks.[17] The expansion over the past decade of AMCs into multihospital chains and primary care practices contributes to their ability to coordinate multiyear clinical trials at various sites. It is far from clear, however, whether they can bring their clinical assets to bear in a cost-effective manner. Nor is it clear that unified ownership is the only mechanism open to AMCs that want to play a central role in clinical investigations. Many of the ancillary facilities and providers that AMCs have acquired specialize in activities in which AMCs have no competitive advantage and no special mission, such as the provision of preventive, primary, and secondary care. Those facilities and providers certainly are complementary assets within the context of clinical trials, but they are not designed to support that function; in such cases, contractual mechanisms appear to be superior to ownership. Nevertheless, it should be reemphasized that today's rush to divest AMCs of community hospitals and primary care practices needs to be tempered with an understanding that the loyalty, commitment, and cooperation of those entities in the management and organization of clinical trials (and, obviously, in clinical teaching) is too important to be sacrificed to overhasty disaffiliations of the type conducted by the physician practice management companies.

Specialty Clinical Services

Academic medical centers will continue to support the most specialized specialists and attract the patients with the most difficult diseases.[18] The mix of formal and informal experimentation that characterizes tertiary care leads to continual improvement in specialty and subspecialty care, although it is doubtful that academic medical centers are an important locus for innovation in methods of primary care. While some AMCs are the sole significant provider in their communities and hence must provide the full range of services, most are in urban areas with many hospitals,

17. Commonwealth Fund (2000); Rettig (2000).
18. Commonwealth Fund (2000).

physicians, and other providers. It briefly appeared that specialty-dominated organizations needed to acquire their own primary care base in order to attract patients. With the retreat of gatekeeping and global capitation, however, it now is evident that primary care physicians, community hospitals, and other ancillary services need not be coordinated in an exclusive fashion with particular specialists, who can continue to attract referrals from all providers. The challenge is to avoid overreacting to contemporary financial difficulties by dumping primary care assets in a manner that will render forming future partnerships difficult.

Conclusion

Despite the contemporary glorification of the entrepreneurial start-up, small and innovative companies often fail while larger organizations succeed, even in the most technologically dynamic industries. Large innovators succeed because they enjoy superior access to specialized and complementary components, production facilities, and distribution channels and because they have marketing know-how and a brand-name reputation. Venture capitalists may supply financing for technology start-ups and provide access to networks of organizational relationships; many of today's largest companies were launched in this manner. But most start-ups eventually are faced with the choice between selling out to a larger and more established competitor or perishing in a vain attempt to remain independent. The advantages of the integrated organization are simply overwhelming.

A sustainable commitment to research requires successful appropriation of the economic benefits of innovation. Successful appropriation, in turn, requires an AMC to have a strategic perspective on which services, facilities, products, and providers it should own, which it should obtain through contract, and which it should leave alone. Too many assets under one roof creates the overextended and unfocused integrated delivery system of yesteryear. Too few complementary assets creates what in the business world is denoted the "hollow corporation," an entity so lean, so stripped of internal capabilities to manufacture, distribute, and service the fruits of its research activities that it starves itself and shrinks into mediocrity. The AMC will never be an entrepreneurial start-up in the exploding market for new laboratory-based and clinical services. It can either remain an overburdened clinical conglomerate or evolve into a disciplined entity with a set of intellectual and physical assets that allow it both to innovate and to appropriate the economic benefits of its innovations.

COMMENT BY
David Blumenthal

As usual, James Robinson has made a provocative and persuasive presentation; it crosses disciplinary boundaries and calls on us to think creatively about existing problems. I agree with his central introductory points about many of the problems and opportunities that academic medical centers face and their origins.

Many AMCs did flock to the integrated delivery system in the early and mid-1990s without giving sufficient thought to how to implement it. Now, some are reflexively reversing strategy, divesting themselves of assets and dis-integrating, again without sufficient thought. Of course, when academic health centers adopted the integrated delivery system, they were not the only organizations to do so; other health care organizations did too. The strategy made a certain amount of sense if one believed that capitation was the wave of the future; it made even more sense for AMCs, because an integrated delivery systems could enable them to fulfill better than ever before certain of their service missions that they had long been accused of neglecting.

For decades before the 1990s, AMCs were criticized for being detached and insulated from their communities, for not caring for the poor populations that lived in their shadow, for being overly involved in specialty care, and for not training physicians to provide primary care. The acquisition of primary care practices, community hospitals, home care agencies, and neighborhood health centers put AMCs right in the middle of their communities in a big way and forced them to provide and teach primary care. In Boston, the big academic centers have poured tens of millions of dollars into community health centers to entice them into clinical alliances. In Memphis, Vanderbilt Medical Center formed an alliance with Meharry Medical College and with a whole series of community health centers. The integration strategy, therefore, was a vehicle for meeting responsibilities that AMCs had long neglected, and their retreat from such alliances threatens to undermine their gains.

Integration seems less necessary from an economic standpoint now because of the retreat of managed care and capitation. If they only had known in advance, AMCs might have avoided some excesses. On Monday, hindsight makes us all astute football tacticians whose advice, applied retrospectively, could have prevented our favorite team from losing on Sunday. But even the well-deserved scorn of Monday morning quarterbacking does not invalidate criticism of how AMCs almost mindlessly implemented the integration strategy. While much can be learned by looking back, the really important questions concern what to do going forward.

In this regard, one of Robinson's most useful contributions is to urge AMCs to think carefully about each of their product lines and how they can be made economically sustainable. Those product lines are teaching, research, and clinical services, the last of which can be divided into multiple product lines, such as high-technology and specialized services, primary and secondary services, and care for vulnerable populations. Robinson uses research as an example of how to think about each of those activities. In some ways, however, his analysis suggests how difficult it may be for AMCs to abandon strategies that enhance revenue but that he finds shortsighted—especially, reliance on government.

The various activities of AMCs are interdependent—often, pursuing one is difficult without the other. Furthermore, achieving excellence in one often requires excellence—or at least competence—in all, or at least several, of them. Robinson acknowledges that AMCs may be the most complex organizations ever created. It was Peter Drucker, I think, who first—or at least most authoritatively—advanced that viewpoint.

How many companies—if we are going to use companies as a model—are expected to be expert in neuroscience and neurobiology, distance education, information technology as it relates to promoting health and monitoring health services, the conduct of clinical trials, the development of decision-support technologies, bone marrow transplants, solid organ transplants, the treatment of burns, and ensuring that primary care of diabetes patients meets accepted guidelines? Yet all are core activities of a modern, premier academic medical center, and each must be sustained with excellence. The challenge of sustaining an AMC becomes oversimplified when one concentrates on a single product line at a time. AMCs are not traditional businesses. Yet, like traditional businesses, they must be good at all of their core activities. Whether such unique organizations can survive in truly competitive markets is an open question.

Even if one focuses just on research, the limits of the business strategy quickly become apparent. If there were a simple business strategy to pursue in that area, the pharmaceutical sector would not be in the state of turmoil that it is now, with numerous pharmaceutical companies going in and out of business. Would we be happy to see the academic medical centers at Harvard, Duke, Yale, UCSF, and Baylor going out of business? Would the public stand for it? That question answers itself, and the answer suggests that if AMCs must play in the business league, they can do so in only limited ways and with substantial protections. One might even argue that the reason that AMCs have contributed so powerfully to health care and even to the biotechnology and pharmaceutical industries—and the reason that many have survived since the seventeenth century, a record matched by few companies—is that they are involved in the production of nonappropriable knowledge: knowledge to which neither they nor any other party can lay exclusive claim. The economic survival of AMCs is much more firmly rooted in their noncommercial contributions than in any business strategies. If they devoted substantially more effort to applied research and development, would they continue to have the natural advantage in basic science that has sustained them in the past?

That question raises a related issue—is it socially beneficial for AMCs to behave like businesses in conducting their research activities? The concern about conflicts of interest that Robinson raises substantially limits AMCs' ability to commercialize their research. AMCs are in some turmoil right now over what kinds of commercial involvements are acceptable for their faculties and for AMCs themselves. I think it likely that several elite AMCs will join Harvard in dramatically restricting the economic interests that investigators are permitted to hold in companies that are funding clinical trials.

Much of the problem with thinking about academic medical centers as businesses is that most people do not really want them to be businesses; they want AMCs to stand apart from and above business and yet contribute to the larger economy. That set of societal expectations, internalized by faculty of AMCs themselves, will always impose limits on using economic analogies and the advice of the Boston Consulting Groups and McKinseys of the world. Those business consultants, after all, bear some responsibility for having gotten academic medical centers into their current predicament—and now are charging generous fees for advice on how to get them out of it.

These conflicts will always dog academic medical centers. While it is important for AMCs to be disciplined and to think through the pros and cons of alternative business strategies, as Robinson suggests, it will always be very hard for them to be disciplined about multiple missions and the production of joint products. And, unfortunately, pressure to make substantial amounts of money will continue to threaten to delegitimize them as institutions.

COMMENT BY
Spencer Foreman

Medical centers often can help themselves, and the experience of the Montefiore Medical Center can be used to support that assertion. I first will describe the environment in which Montefiore operates and how the center is organized; then I will describe certain specifics of our operations, with particular emphasis on strategies that we have employed to confront challenges common to many academic medical centers. I conclude with an assessment of how well the strategies have served us.

Montefiore is located in the Bronx, which has a population of 1.2 million, composed mostly of minorities; African Americans make up 38 percent of the population and Hispanics 42 percent. The population is quite young; nearly one-third of residents are under 18, compared with 23 percent in New York City and 25 percent in New York State. Forty-three percent of the children in the Bronx live in poverty. Teenage mothers account for 14.2 percent of births, a higher proportion than is found anywhere else in New York State. Mortality rates are higher than in the rest of New York City and exceed the state average.

Montefiore has an integrated delivery system comprising two hospitals, primary and specialty care facilities, and a system of post–acute care providers. It also includes a home health care business, a skilled nursing facility, and a rehabilitation center. The 2000 operating budget was $1.235 billion, most from the hospital; $137 million came from faculty practice, $41 million from research and contracts, and $65 million from an independent practice association (IPA). Montefiore had a total of 1.6 million outpatient visits in 2000 and anticipates 1.8 million in 2001. The center is the university hospital and academic medical center for the Albert Einstein College of Medicine. Montefiore handles half of Einstein's clerkships and 800 residents and fellows.

In recent years, Montefiore has faced the same challenges confronting most other medical centers—declining hospital admission rates, increasing local and regional competition, utilization limits, and prices that have risen less than costs. Montefiore came up with a dual strategy to face those challenges, one for expanding business and another for accepting and managing risk. The growth strategy had three major components: to develop a feeder network; to enhance specialty referrals; and to integrate the delivery system. The risk strategy seeks eventually to handle full-risk arrangements. Before Montefiore could adopt those strategies, we had to develop the requisite infrastructure, including facilities, information systems, and an independent practice association.

Throughout the process, Monetiore applied seven strategic principles: to focus on *its* assets and *its* environment in developing its own strategy, rather than to look to other organizations for cues; to build to its own strengths; to fill *real* needs; to establish measurable objectives; to avoid acquiring liabilities (that is, to avoid new affiliations with other institutions and their corresponding sets of new problems); to jettison previous bad decisions; and, finally, to stay focused on the strategy to make sure that the main thing stays the main thing.

The application of these principles to the primary care practices can serve as an example of our strategy. To foster growth, we sought to capitalize on Montefiore's strong community reputation; accordingly, we labeled every facility a *Montefiore* facility and operated all facilities under uniform policies. We acquired practices only to replace physicians. We strove to minimize unavoidable operating losses at each site. The core principle in our primary care strategy, however, was to develop methods of capturing spin-off business.

In 1986, before we began pursuing the strategies outlined above, we had four ambulatory care sites. Now we have thirty, located all over the Bronx and up to mid-Westchester. In ten years, we have added 325,000 square feet of primary care space in the community, plus twelve school sites and six mobile units. Our staff of salaried, full-time primary care physicians has increased from sixty to about 260.

The individual primary care offices lost $24 million in 1998 but generated about 10,000 admissions for the hospital. Those admissions in turn generated about $40 million in hospital revenue beyond patient care costs, which amply repaid the initial loss of about $2,400 per admission. This year, we expect the primary care offices to generate 17,000 admissions and the loss in primary cost facilities per admission to be about $1,000. We anticipate that those patients will generate about $70 million in hospital revenues over costs, without counting the revenue to the faculty practice.

We sought to build faculty practice facilities that were convenient for both the primary care network and the community. Accordingly, we placed major facilities on each campus, so that they could easily become hubs and support our whole feeder system. We also placed facilities in the community to make access more convenient for patients. The investment was significant—including 412,000 square feet of specialty space.

The second part of our strategy was to develop a method for assuming full-risk assessment and management capabilities. That step was important because the Bronx has both a high percentage of families with low cash incomes and a strong tradition of HMO use. HMOs were penetrating very quickly, and it was clear that if Montefiore existed simply as an end-supplier of services it would not survive. As an academic medical center, its costs would be too high to be competitive. Furthermore, as a service vendor to an HMO, it would assume all downside risk without capturing any upside potential.

Our approach was to establish a provider-sponsored, risk-bearing independent practice association (IPA). We developed a strategic partnership with insurers, becoming a reinsurer or subcontractor; we agreed to give them a portion of our profit, and they agreed to give us full-risk arrangements. The insurance companies agreed because Montefiore's control of the market generated substantial leveraging power. We threatened to stay out of their network if they refused to cooperate—and in the Bronx, if you don't do business with Montefiore, you don't do business.

Montefiore began in 1999 with about 65,000 contracts. By 2000, when we took on all of the members of the Health Insurance Plan of New York living in the Bronx and Westchester, we had about 170,000 full-risk contracts. The goal for 2005 is 325,000 contracts. The 170,000 contracts in 2000 generated $300 million in revenue, a substantial chunk of our operating budget.

Between 1993 and 2000 Montefiore made capital investments totaling $691 million: $438 million (63 percent) for acute care infrastructure; $176 million (26 percent) for the ambulatory and network system; and $77 million (11 percent) to develop information technologies. Those investments were financed partly from depreciation, partly from accumulated cash, and partly from fund raising, but primarily from debt.

The capital investments doubled Montefiore's ambulatory patient activity from 800,000 visits in 1993 to 1.6 million in 2000. Adult discharges increased from 38,500 in 1990 to 51,000 in 2000. Average length of stay plummeted from 9.7 days in 1990 to 5.6 days in 2000. In addition, cost per admission in 1999 was 16 percent lower than in 1994.

Between 1995 and 1999, Montefiore's share of total patient discharges in the Bronx rose from 17 percent to 23 percent. By now, that share is probably closer to 25 percent, because our HIP contract was arranged after 1999. Montefiore's gains came not at the expense of its top five competitors, whose shares remained about the same, but from the remaining competitors. Put differently, Montefiore's growth came at the expense of occasional, rather than major, providers.

Growth has not translated into similar increases in profit. The sizeable increase in patient care revenue between 1993 to 1999 produced only modest amounts of net income. When input costs rise and prices cannot be raised to cover the incremental costs, the only way to cover the short-fall is to increase the volume of services—provided that the incremental revenue from those services exceed their incremental cost. Without the increase in patients served, however, Montefiore would likely have suffered serious losses.

COMMENT BY
Edward Miller

In his examination of the economics of innovation in health care, James Robinson points clearly to factors that he believes would lead to the success of academic medical centers. Specifically, he states that the keys to success are focus, transparency, accountability, sensible incentives, and speedy response. I believe not only that he is correct, but also that abundant evidence supports his view.

I will examine each of those keys, drawing on my experience to show how they have helped Johns Hopkins Medicine to remain financially stable and productive in research while continuing to meet its educational goals. As Robinson points out, the clinical enterprise has almost engulfed academic medical centers, leaving research and education behind; one reason has been the lack of sufficient transparency and accountability within the clinical enterprise for its adequate management. While managed care has had a strong effect on the financial well-being of AMCs, it is not solely responsible for the financial problems with which Johns Hopkins and other medical centers have had to grapple, nor do the facts that AMCs care for a disproportionate share of the poor or poorly insured and that training is costly fully explain their financial difficulties. Our measures of the cost of delivering care were poor. Contracts with managed care groups often were undertaken simply to boost volume; the adage "We lose on every sale but we make it up on volume" was not too far from reality. Administrators of many large institutions feared that they would have no patients if they did not accept capitated contracts. However, without reliable and timely data, no improvement in cost control could be made.

Johns Hopkins Medicine adopted a policy of transparency and accountability not only for professional fees but also for hospital fees. Each department director was held accountable for the bottom line. We instituted a system that revealed all monthly revenues and expenses generated by a department so that the director could allocate resources more wisely. Similarly, on the hospital side we put in place a "contribution margin" plan that displayed for directors the hospital expenses and—even more important—the hospital income generated by the patients for whom they were responsible. Having both the school of medicine and the hospital component under the control of the directors allowed for a new sense of accountability and at the same time made information transparent across departments.

The Clinical Practice Association (CPA) was reorganized to include the faculty at large as well as department chairs. That reform made the entire staff accountable and meant that they had a sense of ownership in the effective operation and financial health not only of separate practices but also of the hospital and the university.

Robinson also points out that incentives are necessary for the achievement of goals. We have used incentives very broadly throughout Johns Hopkins Medicine. Personal incentives are built into the salary structure, and performance criteria determine part of each salary. We have quantitative measures of performance for each department, and the incentive payment for the director is based on the performance of the department. Hospital units that perform extremely well receive extra bonuses. Divisions or departments that have exceeded expectations receive additional resources that they can use to establish new programs. The incentive system has been an effective way to change the culture of Johns Hopkins Medicine and to align the objectives of the hospital and the school of medicine.

Robinson notes that AMCs must respond speedily to challenges and opportunities if they are to be effective. Certainly rapid responses are required in a rapidly changing clinical world, but the same could be said of the areas of research and education. One has only to look at the Internet and its effect on education to understand the truth of that observation. Similarly, human genome and stem cell research also require rapid decisionmaking. To respond to that challenge, in 1997 the board of trustees of the Johns Hopkins Hospital and the Johns Hopkins University decided to create Johns Hopkins Medicine, bringing the hospital and health system together with the school of medicine and designating one person to speak for both, the dean/CEO. One person now can speak with one voice for the entire enterprise and respond speedily to issues, whether they concern the clinical practice, research, or education. Since the implementation of that change, I believe we have been able to respond both rapidly and strategically. The formation of Johns Hopkins Medicine also stimulated the board of trustees to think globally across Johns Hopkins Medicine. In the past, trustees concentrated either on hospital functions or research functions. Now they view the entire enterprise as their responsibility and examine the importance of research to the clinical operation.

According to Robinson, focusing on a few important large issues is a major key for success. Four years ago Johns Hopkins Medicine focused on the clinical enterprise. We decided that service was our top priority and that the best way to attract patients was to deliver the best possible medical care, which we defined as taking care of the needs of both patients and their families. Without buying practices, we developed relationships with physicians that made it easier for them to refer patients to us and helped them to get timely responses to their referrals. We decided not to take contracts on which we would lose money, even if that meant that we had to shrink. What we found, however, was that our patients became our advocates and that the managed care companies needed to have us in their panel for them to remain competitive.

We understood that we could probably compete effectively with community hospitals, but we realized that we would not be different from them if we focused only on clinical care; what made us different is innovation. We have to innovate if we are to stay in the lead, whether we are developing new drugs and treatments, finding new ways to use the Internet, developing small molecules to understand how cells function, applying findings from the human genome project, or devising biomechanical devices to make people better. Our position is not qualitatively different from that of a pharmaceutical house that must have a pipeline of new compounds ready to bring to market.

We therefore focused on our strengths—in this case, research. As the institution with more NIH grants than any other, we were confident that we could sustain quality, so we focused on those areas in which we thought we could make the most impact: oncology, genetics, neuroscience, and cell engineering. We had many of the pieces in place already, and we were able to organize them coherently to drive the scientific agenda for Johns

Hopkins Medicine, assisted not only by NIH grants but also by very large gifts from private donors. And we are counting on continued philanthropic support. Over the next ten years, roughly $10 trillion dollars will pass from one generation to the next. It is vital for the future health of academic medical centers that some of those dollars flow to them.

AMCs have gone through some difficult times, and they will again in the future. However, I believe that success can be achieved by remaining focused and making sure that there is transparency and accountability, coupled with meaningful incentives. AMCs will have many opportunities: they may include a developing an e-health initiative or a new biomedical device that transforms the care of thousands of people. We all understand that only fundamental changes in treatment will cause significant changes in the cost of health care. A generation ago streptomycin permitted the rapid cure of patients with tuberculosis who theretofore had remained in sanatoriums for years. Similar breakthroughs in the future will alter the face of medicine. Some will raise costs, others will lower costs, but it is only through innovation that we will be able to make significant changes.

General Discussion

Samuel Hellman commented that academic medical centers traditionally have found it difficult to capture the economic benefits of their own innovations; although many hospitals have tried, they have not succeeded as well as have large corporations. Hellman proposed a research project to investigate where and by whom major technological discoveries have been made and where and by whom the discoveries subsequently were commercialized. He expressed the view that large corporations may reap most of the rewards, with very little return to the innovators. Allen Dobson noted that it is difficult to appropriate products that have social benefits. With certain discoveries, such as the stent, there are conflicts of interest in not sharing.

Peter Van Etten expressed the view that appropriation is not really necessary, because the federal government pays $20 billion a year to support research. Kenneth Shine observed that even with government funding, research is very costly; academic medical centers must supplement every dollar of a grant from the National Institutes of Health with 20 to 25 cents of their own funds. Lawrence Lewin noted that unsponsored faculty research is another important issue for AMCs to address. While unsponsored research produces undoubted benefits, the flexibility granted to senior faculty through the tenure system also creates significant fixed costs. Shine pointed out that academic medical centers must do more than research to stay in business, including provide relatively routine patient care, and that their operations must be well managed, partly to support high-tech pursuits.

Lewin rejected the notion that the integrated delivery system (IDS) is an unambiguously failed strategy. He argued that many of the failures have resulted not from the strategy itself, but from rushed implementation of the strategy. James Robinson noted that both the IDS and divestment strategies could be oversold, suggesting that AMCs identify which activities are complements and eliminate those that are not.

Lewin also commented that many academic medical centers are not effectively exploiting philanthropic giving as a source of revenue. In his view, philanthropy should be used not only to build endowments but also to support current operations. Spencer Foreman agreed that philanthropic support is essential to sustaining the academic enterprise but argued that it should be used to elicit large contributions for special purposes, rather than for day-to-day operations. Henry Aaron noted that the proposed repeal of the estate and gift tax poses a major threat to charitable giving.

Joseph Newhouse observed that the lack of standardized accounting methods as well as some organizations' failure to divulge information is a source of much of the difficulty in understanding the financial state of academic medical centers. He wondered whether the Financial Accounting Standards Board could take action to establish some type of standard for accounting among AMCs.

Van Etten agreed with Robinson that academic medical centers must learn how to operate effectively within a competitive environment, but he questioned whether they have to appropriate the benefits of their own innovations. He noted that competitive advantage results not from copying but from differentiation; the challenge for academic medicine is to overcome obstacles in the academic culture that prevent them from realizing the benefits of differentiation. Van Etten suggested that rather than trying to look like ordinary businesses, AMCs should try to take advantage of the unique attribute of the academic medical center—the ability to provide services that other providers cannot.

Bruce Vladeck wondered which model is most appropriate for academic medical centers. He said that he is continually struck by how fundamentally academic AMCs are; for that reason, the operations of other health care providers are not really a relevant reference point. The university model is not necessarily appropriate either, because most customers of universities—specifically, students—can find means to pay for their services, while two-thirds of inpatient medical surgical patients cannot afford to pay. Vladeck reminded the conferees that the government is the principal purchaser of academic health centers' services and that a principal economic actor in academic health centers are tenured faculty, whose behavior is unlike that of almost all other employees. The AMC is not a typical business because payments come overwhelmingly from third-party payers and government; ordinary market incentives are not effective in that type of situation. Herbert Pardes concurred that the academic medical center is a functionally unique entity in which the free operation of market incentives may interfere with the achievement of the institution's basic mission, particularly since most of its customers cannot pay their bills directly.

Nancy Kane commented that through the lens of its finances, Foreman's hospital does not appear to be particularly successful. Montefiore has grown substantially but at the expense of accruing substantial debt and achieving only break-even status at best. She suggested that perhaps ordinary financial tests are inappropriate for evaluating medical centers. Foreman replied that he has come to measure success not against the optimal but against the possible and that in that sense his institution is a huge success.

David Blumenthal agreed that academic medical centers cannot be evaluated purely as another business. Before one can decide whether losing the bottom 25 percent of institutions is acceptable, one must decide what the goals of academic medical centers are. What levels of research would we like to conduct? How many people do we want to train? What level of specialized service do we want to sustain? Dobson commented that the challenge facing AMCs is a tough one. Their costs are 10 to 30 percent higher than those of community hospitals. The reasons for the cost difference may well be legitimate, but that difference still makes it hard for AMCs to compete.

Robinson observed that the public does not seem willing to finance all of the activities that AMC faculty and managers would like to undertake. The public is willing to provide some support, Robinson noted, but only if AMCs are seen as making a strong effort to find their own resources, to demonstrate solid management, and to come close to being self-sustaining—in short, to perform well in both the market place and the political arena.

References

Blumenthal, David, Joel S. Weissman, and Peter F. Griner. 1999. "Academic Health Centers on the Front Lines: Survival Strategies in Highly Competitive Markets." *Academic Medicine* 74 (9): 1038–49.

Cohen, Wesley M., and Richard C. Levin. 1989. "Empirical Studies of Innovation and Market Structure." In *Handbook of Industrial Organization*, vol. 2, edited by Richard Schmalensee and Richard D. Willig, 1060–98. Amsterdam: Elsevier Science Publishers.

Cohen, Stephen, and John Zysman. 1987. *Manufacturing Matters: The Myth of the Post-Industrial Economy.* New York: Basic Books.

Commonwealth Fund. 1999. *From Bench to Bedside: Preserving the Research Mission of Academic Health Centers.* New York.

———. 2000. *Health Care at the Cutting Edge: The Role of Academic Health Centers in the Provision of Specialty Care.* New York.

Dosi, Giovanni. 1988. "Sources, Procedures, and Microeconomic Effects of Innovation." *Journal of Economic Literature* 26: 1120–71.

Feinstein, Adam T., and Joshua R. Raskin. 2000. *Health Care Facilities Outlook and Guidebook.* New York: Lehman Brothers.

Goldstein, L., and others. 2000. *Not-for-Profit Health Care: 2000 Outlook and Medians.* New York: Moody's Investors Service.

Griner, Paul, and David Blumenthal. 1998. "Reforming the Structure and Management of Academic Medical Centers: Case Studies of Ten Institutions." *Academic Medicine* 73 (7): 818–25.

Heller, Michael A., and Rebecca S. Eisenberg. 1998. "Can Patents Deter Innovation? The Anticommons in Biomedical Research." *Science* 280: 698–701.

Hunter, David. 2000. *Hunterbert's Twelve-Step Performance Improvement Program.* Presentation to Harvard School of Public Health, Boston, November 2.

Kenney, Martin. 1986. *Biotechnology: The University-Industrial Complex.* New Haven, Conn.: Yale University Press.

Martin, J. B., and D. K. Kasper. 2000. "In Whose Best Interest? Breaching the Academic-Industrial Wall." *New England Journal of Medicine* 343 (22): 1646–49.

Nelson, Richard R. 1990. "Capitalism as an Engine of Progress." *Research Policy* 19: 193–214.

Pavitt, Keith. 1984. "Sectoral Patterns of Technical Change: Towards a Taxonomy and a Theory." *Research Policy* 13: 343–73.

Pisano, Gary. 1991. "The Governance of Innovation: Vertical Integration and Collaborative Arrangements in the Biotechnology Industry." *Research Policy* 20: 237–49.

Powell, Walter. 1987. "Hybrid Organizational Arrangements: New Form or Transitional Development?" *California Management Review* 29: 67–87.

Rettig, Richard. 2000. "The Industrialization of Clinical Research." *Health Affairs* 19 (2): 129–46.

Schumpeter, Joseph A. 1962. *Capitalism, Socialism, and Democracy* (originally published 1942). New York: Harper Torchbooks.

Shapiro, Carl, and Hal R. Varian. 1999. *Information Rules: A Strategic Guide to the Network Economy.* Cambridge, Mass.: Harvard Business School Press.

Teece, David J. 1992. "Competition, Cooperation, and Innovation." *Journal of Economic Behavior and Organization* 18 (1): 1–25.

———. 1998. "Capturing Value from Knowledge Assets: The New Economy, Markets for Know-How, and Intangible Assets." *California Management Review* 40 (3): 55–79.

———. 1986. "Profiting from Technological Innovation: Implications for Integration, Collaboration, Licensing, and Public Policy." *Research Policy* 15: 285–305.

Zuckerman, L., J. Rodgers, and T. Goode. 2000. *An Overview of Academic Medical Centers.* Standard & Poor's Public Finance Department.

CHAPTER FOUR

Politically Feasible and Practical Public Policies to Help Academic Medical Centers

Lawrence S. Lewin

The three major missions of academic medical centers are to educate the health care work force; engage in basic and clinical research in the life sciences; and provide advanced specialty care and care for uninsured and underserved patients. This chapter outlines a range of politically feasible and practical public policies to help academic medical centers to carry out those missions and to retain their position as leaders in the U.S. health care system. Before proposing solutions, however, one should first identify the problem. Accordingly, I identify problems and propose solutions in each mission area. One additional issue merits particular mention—how federal policies can advance adoption by AMCs of information technology, which is becoming increasingly important to their success.

Setting the Context

Because they have multiple, intertwined missions, AMCs are complex institutions. Some of the services they provide are joint products—for example, training clinicians is a byproduct of clinical care—making it almost impossible to measure accurately the costs of many AMC activities. That fact is especially troublesome when the major purchaser of AMCs' products and services—the federal government—prefers to pay on the basis of cost rather than market price. Not surprisingly then, much of public policy with respect to AMCs continues to be mired in the economic complexities of cost finding. Although payment issues are important, I focus less on such technical issues than on broader issues affecting AMCs.

AMCs' efforts to provide education, perform research, and offer indigent care typically serve national goals, and AMCs receive considerable reimbursement from the federal government in each area. But because rules regarding reimbursement and payment are established by different federal programs designed and funded by various congressional committees, they are uncoordinated. For example, Medicare payments for direct and indirect medical education and Medicare disproportionate share hospital (DSH) reimbursements fall under the aegis of the congressionally mandated Medicare Payment Advisory Commission (MedPAC). Medicare, however, accounts for only about one-third of AMCs' net patient revenues. Subsidies associated with Medicaid, third-party payments, and other payments for uncompensated care are determined by other government and private sector entities on both the national and state level. (The federal government also pays for many services and products indirectly because funds are imprecisely applied; in such cases, those funds may end up supporting activities that the government did not intend to support.)

Despite the financial stresses experienced in recent years, especially in the aftermath of the Balanced Budget Act of 1997, AMCs *overall* remain robust institutions, respected in their communities and performing vital national functions. Some, however, are clearly in financial jeopardy. Others, as Nancy Kane's findings suggest (see chapter 2), may be less endangered than they appear, especially when all components of the AMC are explored.

But the trends are not encouraging, especially for institutions that face heavy costs for indigent care. If AMCs continue to bear that burden, they will remain vulnerable to competition from other hospitals that skim the cream off the top by favoring insured patients.[1] In a price-competitive market, the more that public policy continues to rely on the capacity of AMCs to finance care for the indigent and the uninsured by levying charges that exceed the cost of care on the well-insured, the greater the likelihood that AMCs and other mission-driven institutions will be in financial trouble, that mission commitments will be eroded, or—most likely—both.

1. Gbadebo and Reinhardt (2001).

Three Underlying Problems

AMCs face three problems that call for public policy action; solutions to all three have remained elusive. That the first problem—how to finance care for the indigent—would be greatly ameliorated if health insurance coverage were universal requires little elaboration. The failure of the Clinton Health Plan and the current focus on incremental reform reduce the likelihood of major extensions of health insurance coverage to close to zero, at least in the short term. To be sure, some organizations currently are developing proposals that attempt to achieve near-universal coverage through the expansion of existing programs. For example, "A 2020 Vision for American Health Care," a proposal developed under the auspices of the Commonwealth Fund, outlines a new and rather bold plan for achieving such a goal.[2] Another approach, developed under the auspices of the Robert Wood Johnson Foundation and referred to as the "Strange Bedfellows Proposal," brings together the Health Insurance Association of America, Families U.S.A., and the American Hospital Association behind an incremental approach that, at best, would reduce the ranks of the uninsured by about 6 million people.[3] But these approaches have generated little support in Congress, largely because program expansions are unlikely given its preoccupation with tax reduction.

The second underlying problem is an excess of medical schools, especially in urban areas such as New York City, Philadelphia, and Chicago. Although the United States may not be producing too many physicians, fewer schools probably could educate the same number of physicians at lower cost and improve not only the ability of the remaining institutions to survive but also to invest in needed infrastructure improvements, modernized teaching programs, and information technology.

Although the obstacles to closing, merging, or even downsizing medical schools are daunting, public policy could encourage consolidation in a number of ways. More restrictive reimbursement rules would challenge all institutions, allowing only the fittest to survive. Policymakers should be concerned, however, about what may be lost when weak institutions vanish—for example, when a medical school is a major provider of training for underrepresented minorities or the sole source of care for

2. Davis, Schoen, and Schoenbaum (2000).
3. Kahn and Pollack (2001).

underinsured populations. Unfortunately, it is difficult to forecast the full range of consequences of such a policy. More positive incentives for consolidation include dealing flexibly with the rigid requirements of many debt instruments; favorable terms for transferring or reducing the number of medical residents; and loans to finance the closure of marginal institutions. However, public policy may not be able to do anything about what I have found to be the most serious obstacles to consolidation—institutional history, the drive toward self-preservation, and powerful egos.

The third problem is the conflict between efforts to expose health care providers to the economic discipline of the market and continuing reliance on implicit cross-subsidies that enable AMCs to provide "public goods" that in other sectors usually are provided by the government. The best example is the provision of health care to indigent patients. Public hospitals and clinics, together with urban and many rural teaching hospitals, are expected to provide care to the uninsured financed by Medicaid and a variety of other federal, state, and local programs or by "profits" realized from charging privately insured patients more than the cost of care. More than half of all hospital uncompensated care is delivered by private hospitals through such cost shifting.[4] This system worked reasonably well when businesses, governments, and other purchasers of health care services were less price conscious than they are today and when reimbursement was based mainly on costs or charges. Today's increasingly price-competitive and discount-oriented market is rapidly eroding cross-subsidies, creating strong incentives for hospitals to abandon care for the poor and other services for which there is inadequate or no payment. AMCs appear to be resisting those incentives. They have a historical commitment to indigent care; in addition, they need indigent cases for their teaching programs. Federal and state governments assist institutions in their care of poor patients through such policies as disproportionate share hospital payments. But in many states DSH funds are diverted to hospitals that serve relatively few poor or uninsured patients. Some states use DSH funds for non–health-related services.[5]

Education

The major educational problems confronting AMCs are pedagogical and curricular in nature. Too many topics need to be taught in a limited pe-

---

4. Mann and others (1997).
5. Ku and Coughlin (1995).

riod. At the same time, increasingly important areas such as nutrition, human sexuality, and medical safety are not adequately addressed. In addition, AMCs need to modernize their facilities, manage their resources better, and improve the integration of education and clinical care. Finally, AMCs should enhance interdisciplinary learning and explore new pedagogical techniques.

To some extent, National Institutes of Health (NIH) grants are helping to promote integrated, multidisciplinary operations within AMCs, but the impact of NIH grants is greater on research than on education and training. As the practice of medicine shifts from inpatient to outpatient care, schools of medicine are seeking new training sites, with a particular focus on primary care. That shift requires AMCs to have faculty practitioners who can offer clinical instruction at community-based sites so that students can learn primary and ambulatory specialty care under faculty supervision. The added costs and supervisory problems associated with these new requirements all pose sizable challenges. At the same time that the practice of community medicine is growing, so too is the need for laboratory scientists with both medical training and advanced education in a scientific discipline. Research into the fundamental causes and treatment of disease requires increasing numbers of medical doctors with Ph.D. degrees, and AMCs will have to train them. Yet financial pressures on newly minted physicians and the financial lure of clinical practice have dimmed the appeal to medical doctors of advanced training in non-medical disciplines.

The future of nursing represents another major challenge. Recent evidence indicates that the United States is experiencing yet another potentially severe shortage of nurses. Past shortages were across the board, arising when a boom economy lured nurses into other activities; the current shortage appears to be more enduring, more complex, and potentially more harmful. It is being felt most keenly in high-skill areas such as critical care and in emergency and operating rooms. Furthermore, the nursing work force is aging more rapidly than the overall population. The proportion of registered nurses age 35 and younger fell from 40 percent in 1980 to 18 percent today; the average age of nurses now is more than 43 years.[6] A shortage of nurse educators also has been reported, particularly of faculty prepared to train nurses to provide care in community settings.

6. Health Resources and Services Administration (2001).

Building an adequate nursing work force for the future may require review of the barriers to licensing and practice that some states retain, including denying nurses the authority to prescribe drugs, denying reimbursement to nurses for services that they are well qualified to provide, and excluding nurses from independent practice. Many of these laws and limitations represent outdated "protectionism" for physicians, and they preclude opportunities to improve productivity.

The first step in dealing with nursing and other educational problems is to recognize that the problems exist. I believe a national conference on the future of nursing, hosted by an independent group such as the Institute of Medicine, could help sort out the myriad and highly divisive issues not only between the practice of medicine and nursing, but also within nursing. Such a conference should examine the various levels of education required to meet future demand for nurses, the role and support of foreign-born and foreign-educated nurses, strategies for increasing the supply of both nurses and nurse educators, and ways to modify state licensing policies to fairly address the problem of practice limitations.

Solutions to pedagogical problems are available. The first is to increase funding for faculty research on educational methods. Few medical schools do formal research on how to teach effectively, yet innovation in education merits support as much as do other new technologies. Such inquiries have received little recognition, but they hold great potential. Currently, most educators play a marginal role within the AMC power structure, and many complain that pressure to generate clinical revenue puts increasing pressure on their capacity to prepare for and meet their teaching responsibilities. Greater focus on both teaching and research into educational activities could advance curriculum reform in medical education. Federal government and foundation grants could support and assess promising innovations and fund faculty positions in the educational area.

Second, AMCs individually and as a group should invest in the development of new computer-based systems of learning. Virtual reality models, for example, can dramatically increase the efficiency of medical education, and they may reduce dependence on costly outpatient settings that often are difficult to manage. Such programs are expensive to develop; once developed, however, they can be replicated at relatively low cost. The academic community could share these costs, but modest federal support or cost sharing would be helpful.

Third, financial incentives should be offered to encourage highly qualified students to pursue M.D./Ph.D. degrees.

Research in the Life Sciences

The huge success of U.S. government support of research in the life sciences is indisputable and internationally recognized—support of the human genome project is the most recent stellar example. And the remarkable breakthroughs in radiology and many other areas of practice would not have taken place without federal government support.

AMCs conduct 42 percent of health-related research and development activities in the United States.[7] The rapid increase in NIH extramural research funding has contributed to aggressive growth in the research enterprise of academic medical centers (although the almost manic preoccupation of some institutions with increasing their share of that growth could present cause for worry). To capitalize on the growth in the NIH budget, many academic medical centers are building facilities and incurring other fixed costs, such as that for added tenured faculty. Those commitments represent potential burdens should growth of NIH funding or clinical practice reimbursement falter, especially in a highly constrained fiscal environment.

NIH currently requires grantees to provide approximately 20 percent of the cost of the grants themselves. That cost, coupled with the institutions' need to support some level of "unsponsored" research—such as the time required by faculty to prepare grants proposals or preliminary research to develop "fundable" hypotheses—can divert resources from support for education and clinical services.

Unfortunately, as Peter Van Etten has observed, current accounting practices have made it very difficult for both AMCs themselves and the government to understand how much various activities really cost. Current work by the Association of American Medical Colleges (AAMC) in mission accounting and by the University HealthCare Consortium (UHC) in funds flow analysis may shed some light on those questions. At present, however, it is hard to know whether federal payments for research are adequate or fair. Whatever the outcome, some leaders of academic medical centers have come to recognize that supporting a rapidly growing research enterprise while meeting NIH's cost-sharing requirements puts so much financial pressure on educational funding that education programs are being shortchanged. It may prove especially difficult for some private medical schools, especially those without significant endowments, to meet new space requirements and to compete for high-cost faculty.

7. Commonwealth Fund (1997, p. 24).

A case can be made, however, for cooperative funding of research by NIH. Some research has produced lucrative commercial payoffs for AMCs (for example, the development of Gatorade by the University of Florida), but examples of those payoffs are few and their overall benefit to AMCs has not been measured. Furthermore, the pursuit of technology transfer raises ethical problems and may threaten the traditional open communication and disclosure practices so essential to good science.

Another reported problem stems from the low NIH salary cap for fellowships—in the mid $30,000s range—that discourage U.S.-educated students from accepting them. Although the cohort of postdoctoral fellows is large—roughly 60,000—a large proportion currently are foreign born or foreign educated. To attract U.S. citizens, AMCs must increase stipends from their own resources. The low salary cap for senior researchers on NIH extramural grants also serves as another way of imposing institutional cost sharing. A similar problem arises in pay for senior professors, who cannot be paid more than $141,000 a year from NIH grants. Salary caps, both for senior investigators on extramural grants and for postdoctoral fellows, should be raised. Current policy is a serious obstacle to recruiting, retaining top investigators, and attracting young Americans to long-term careers in life sciences research.

Whether to maintain cost-sharing requirements for NIH grants and how to reimburse for indirect costs raise both technical problems, such as how to calculate indirect rates, and policy considerations. Is it better to fund existing grantees more fully or to provide more grants? The former policy would direct more funds to a smaller number of institutions, but it would cover all costs. The latter policy would not cover all costs, but it would result in more grants, perhaps increasing the diversity of institutions and programs funded. There is no clear answer to the question of which is the better approach. In making that decision, it would help to know whether NIH grantees receive collateral benefits that have economic value—such as the ability to attract better faculty, residents, and fellows or to obtain more private sector funding—that justify keeping payments below costs. And, if so, what would a fair financial burden on institutions be? On those issues, opinions abound, but analysis is scarce. The issues, however, persist, as funding policies need to be reassessed periodically in light of national research targets and their impact on recipients.

On the question of technology transfer, consideration should be given to the development of a federally sponsored, quasi-governmental venture capital fund. The fund eventually could be financed, at least in part, by equity shares that the federal government would hold in major technology transfer enterprises generated by NIH-funded labs. The federal equity position in any single enterprise may be only 10 to15 percent, but when there are returns, the administering agency could accumulate those returns to fund higher-risk, basic science research, such as the highly successful human genome project.

Provision of Advanced Medical Care and Care for the Underserved

AMCs not only develop and make available advanced systems of medical care but also serve in many communities as a major and dependable source of care for the uninsured and others without access to care. The confluence of these two roles means that indigent care patients serve as teaching cases for medical students and residents. AMCs traditionally have provided services to the uninsured as part of their mission; in addition, the location of many AMCs in poor, inner-city areas makes them a logical site for indigent care. The fact that AMCs provide a disproportionate share of the nation's uncompensated care thus is not surprising, but the financial consequences of that burden are of increasing concern.

First, clinical revenues from insured patients, including Medicare and Medicaid patients, are not adequate to finance indigent care. Medicare diagnosis related groups (DRG) payments are geared to patients with average acuity, but AMCs often serve the sickest patients with the most complicated conditions. Extra payments are available for cases that cost substantially more than average, and while they are helpful, they almost always are inadequate. In addition, in parts of the country with high HMO penetration, managed care plans are siphoning off patients whose cost of care is below average, leaving those with more complex problems to the care of teaching hospitals.[8]

Second, graduate medical education funding for AMCs and other teaching hospitals comes primarily from two special Medicare payments. The first, direct graduate medical education (DGME) payments, cover Medicare's share of costs directly associated with the operation of intern and resident training programs; the amount of payment is determined on a hospital-specific, per-resident basis. Direct costs include salary and fringe benefits for interns, residents, and teaching physicians, along with other

8. Meyer and Blumenthal (1996).

costs that can be directly related to training programs. The second component relates to the so-called indirect costs of graduate medical education (IME), such as the relatively higher costs of patient care in AMCs and teaching hospitals. IME payments were begun in 1980, when Medicare allowed an adjustment to help cover the higher costs per case observed in teaching hospitals. Considerable effort has gone into analyzing what IME payments should be, but no clear conclusions have emerged. In the end, the size of payments always has been a fiscal and policy decision. IME rates have tightened over the years. A more recent problem is that managed care organizations with Medicare or Medicaid contracts collect IME payments but may not use the funds for their intended purpose. According to the Congressional Budget Office, GME funding, not including state Medicaid GME, totaled $7.1 billion in 1998.

A third problem concerns Medicare and Medicaid payments made to hospitals that serve a relatively large volume of low-income patients—so-called disproportionate share hospital (DSH) payments. The Medicaid DSH program was created in 1981 to "take into account the situation of hospitals that serve a disproportionate number of low-income patients with special needs" by making "additional Medicaid payments to those facilities." The law gave states broad flexibility in designing their DSH programs. Consequently there is a great deal of variation in the generosity of those programs, the institutions eligible to receive funds, and the conditions imposed on recipients. In 1998, Medicaid DSH payments to hospitals totaled $15 billion, representing more than 8 percent of Medicaid spending.

The Balanced Budget Act of 1997 called for gradual reductions of and caps on DSH payments, but legislation in 1999 suspended most of the proposed cutbacks. While DSH funding has played a critical role in supporting institutions that provide care for low-income patients, many states use DSH funds to supplement low Medicaid payment rates rather than to support uninsured care.[9] In addition, DSH funds flow through hospitals and virtually exclude payments to ambulatory care providers.

A fourth issue revolves around states' circumvention of federal matching rules to avoid spending extra money themselves, an abuse that has been a well-established source of funding under the Medicaid statutes. In poorer states the federal match can be as high as 80 percent; the average federal match is close to 56 percent.[10] Federal expansion of eligibility for

9. Coughlin, Ku, and Kim (2000).
10. Kaiser Commission on Medicaid and the Uninsured (2001).

Medicaid over recent years, together with healthy state budgets, has encouraged a number of states to significantly broaden eligibility for their Medicaid programs and for the new State Children's Health Insurance Program (SCHIP) in order to reduce the number of uninsured patients. To help finance these expansions, states and municipalities have developed some creative mechanisms for using public and private funds to bring in federal matching dollars. Congress and the U.S. Department of Health and Human Services now are critically assessing some of those practices.

A final set of issues revolves around philanthropy—hospitals' "last resort" for funding indigent care. Overall hospital Medicare margins declined between 1996 and 1999, as Nancy Kane shows (see chapter 2). According to MedPAC, some improvement in margins occurred in 2000.[11] Nevertheless, most observers believe that the margins of most major teaching hospitals will continue to decline. Philanthropy can help these institutions, but only in a limited way. Most philanthropic funding goes to capital projects and highly visible high-technology clinical programs, not to services. Unless the thrust of philanthropy changes, AMCs must depend on payments by government and other payers to cover the cost of services, including the disproportionate provision of expensive specialty care. In that context, the sluggish adjustment of Medicare DRG payments is problematic. Many new and costly drugs and medical devices, even ones that produce improved outcomes and lower costs in the long run, may cost more than the existing DRG payment covers. The fact that it takes many months or even years to update DRG prices puts AMCs and other institutions that are leaders in innovation and clinical care at a disadvantage. Until the DRGs are adjusted, they find themselves underreimbursed by Medicare for new treatments and thereby subject to financial stress.

Many practices and procedures that have the potential to improve health or prevent illness simply are not reimbursed at all, particularly under Medicare's predominantly fee-for-service and procedure-oriented reimbursement system. Payments typically do not rise commensurately with the duration of the physician-patient encounter, thereby reducing doctors' incentives to spend time counseling patients on how to stay healthy.

At the risk of stating the obvious, I will point out that reducing the ranks of the uninsured would make a major dent in the financial difficulties facing academic medical centers. Plans to greatly extend coverage, such as the Vision 2020 Plan, appear to be feasible and practical; nonethe-

11. Medicare Payment Advisory Commission (2001).

less, only tax credits or incremental extensions of coverage seem likely in the near term. The experience to date with SCHIP suggests that incremental steps may be less fruitful than originally estimated. However, the current federal effort to increase enrollment and retention in SCHIP could have a significant payoff, especially if matched by major efforts of private philanthropic foundations.

The DSH programs—especially Medicaid's—need a fresh look. DSH funding should be maintained or expanded. However, the DSH formulas should be designed to take better account of the services provided to uninsured patients and the limited ability of many providers to shift costs to private payers. Eligibility for DSH funding should be broadened to include providers other than hospitals that care for the medically indigent. And rules should ensure that DSH funds are used primarily for indigent care, not to supplement Medicaid payments.

The MedPAC proposal to consolidate support of graduate medical education into a single payment is attractive but debatable. The MedPAC proposal is preferable to making annual appropriations, especially for indirect medical education costs, because the need for annual approval would expose the program to unpredictable and unnecessary political and fiscal risk. But debate must also address the problem of ensuring that the funds are preserved for their intended purpose. The special trust fund for GME proposed by the AAMC and others should be given serious consideration.

New Medicare reimbursement policies need to be developed, including within Medicare+Choice, to encourage payment of physicians not only for face-to-face encounters but also for contacts through the Internet and other forms of distance communication, such as telephone consultations. These alternatives are particularly promising as educational tools and in monitoring chronically ill, infirm, and homebound patients.

Various technical improvements in Medicare and Medicaid would assist AMCs and are overdue. HCFA, in conjunction with the Agency for Healthcare Research and Quality and MedPAC, should update DRG prices more rapidly than is now done when there is compelling evidence that more costly, advanced clinical methods or preventive measures result in improved outcomes. Risk-adjustment mechanisms for Medicare and Medicaid do not adequately compensate hospitals for the added costs of treating very sick patients. Unless and until more accurate adjustments can be developed, Congress should give serious consideration to a national reinsurance pool, perhaps administered by Medicare to reduce current incentives for hospitals to avoid sicker patients.

Telecommunications Technologies

Information and telecommunications technologies will have a powerful influence on the evolution of all aspects of health care and the health sciences. Some academic medical centers and other centers of advanced life sciences research already have made extensive use of bioinformatics, a new interdisciplinary field connecting genomics, the biological sciences, computational methods, and engineering.[12] Advanced research in genomics, proteomics, molecular biology, nanotechnologies, and imaging rely heavily on high-speed, large-memory supercomputers and on the talents and skills of specialists in computer sciences and in computational biology.

Unfortunately, application of informatics to the management of health care systems has lagged far behind its application in other industries. Because health care has failed to exploit currently available information and telecommunications technologies, it has foregone potentially valuable opportunities, such as those to reduce the cost of and time spent on claims filing, processing, and payment; to reduce unexplained variations in clinical care; to identify, analyze, and reduce medical errors, especially in the management of prescription drugs; to adopt physician-order entry systems to reduce errors and provide for immediate feedback to physicians and other caregivers; to use wireless communications for online, real-time monitoring of patient condition and for patient reporting of changes in status, especially for chronic illness; and to engage patients in self-management of their health.

While full exploitation of the potential benefits of new technologies depends on action by all of the major players in the health care industry, federal leadership—which has not, by and large, been forthcoming in recent years[13]—has an important role to play. The federal government, through Medicare and Medicaid payment provisions, could help develop and implement industrywide standards, definitions, and formats. Conditions of participation in those payment programs could include a requirement for physician-order entry protocols; standardized systems of patient identifiers; electronic patient records; and workable coding systems to protect patient confidentiality. The federal government also could establish a standardized coding and billing form for use by all private insurers, somewhat akin to Medicare's Uniform Billing Form UB-82; such a form would solve one of the more vexing and costly problems faced by both hospitals

12. *New York Times*, March 25, 2001.
13. Shortliffe (2000).

and physicians—the use of different billing formats and review standards by health plans. Finally, given the enormous costs and risks associated with adopting new information systems, the government should liberalize rules for how reimbursement of those costs can be built into rates; it might also finance demonstration projects and systems development efforts.

Final Observations

Some of the policy proposals I have suggested would require additional federal funding, but many would not. Clarification of existing policies would cost little, but it would assist AMCs. In some significant areas, such as Medicaid DSH funding, unclear provisions have led to misuse. It also is essential for the federal government to recognize that it has a major and pivotal role to play in the adoption of new technologies, both in establishing standards and, in some cases, underwriting the costs. In the end, however, many of the improvements needed must come from the academic medical centers themselves.

COMMENT BY
Robert Dickler

Lawrence Lewin has done an excellent job of outlining problems in academic medicine and potential public policy solutions to those problems. I will first comment and expand on some of his observations and then articulate a somewhat broader policy perspective.

First, Lewin suggested that there are too many medical schools. We could certainly debate the validity of that conclusion for the nation, but there may well be too many medical schools in some urban areas or other locations. We should remember, as Lewin points out, that too many medical schools does not necessarily mean too many medical students. Instead of considering the number of medical schools, we should think about whether we are training too many, too few, or the right number of students.

The current evidence on that question is in many ways contradictory. The number of applicants to medical schools has fallen, but there is pressure to expand the number of medical students, evidenced by several new osteopathic schools and a new medical school being developed in Florida. Some indicators suggest that we have too few openings in U.S. medical schools.

Second, it is important to distinguish between undergraduate and graduate medical education; some issues apply to both, but in general their problems differ. Medical schools have undertaken substantial changes in the undergraduate curriculum, using, for example, innovative information-based technologies. The September 2000 supplement of the journal *Academic Medicine* summarizes those changes. Graduate medical education, through the efforts of the Accreditation Council for Graduate Medical Education, the Association of American Medical Colleges, and other organizations, is now focused on developing core curriculum content and outcome measures of competency for MDs completing their residency program. Given those initiatives, it is not clear to me that government policy or regulatory initiatives related to either undergraduate or graduate medical education would be productive or appropriate except to support pilot or demonstration projects.

Third, Lewin omitted two topics with important public policy implications: student diversity and geographic balance. Current medical school students differ greatly in race, sex, and ethnicity from the physicians now in the workforce, and both differ from the general population. Regarding the number of physicians, many people have commented that the problem is not that there are too many or too few but that they are not in the right places. Those are old issues. Both diversity and distribution have policy implications ranging from affirmative action, to loans and scholarships for medical education, to the systemization of the delivery of health services.

Fourth, I would urge everyone who talks about the funding of graduate medical education through Medicare to recognize that there are two distinct funding streams. One provides some funding for the direct costs of graduate medical education (GME). The other, labeled "indirect medical education," provides resources to cover the differential costs that teaching hospitals incur because they handle more severe cases, perform other distinctive services, and carry out research. Gail Wilensky has discussed the MedPAC proposal to combine those funding streams. But I would urge us to avoid using a general GME label unless that proposal becomes reality. Otherwise, discussions about GME funding typically generate a great deal of confusion.

There also is a tendency to confound two distinct flows of funds to hospitals providing a disproportionate share of indigent care (disproportionate share payments), one from Medicare, the other from Medicaid. They are quite different in many ways, and any proposed policy changes need to take those differences into account. The purpose of the transfers is not to subsidize the other missions of academic medicine by supporting indigent care; the simple fact is that many teaching hospitals provide such care. The two sources of funding are linked because of the history and location of many teaching hospitals. There was a deliberate effort to try to"delink" them when the original Medicare disproportionate share hospital payments were carved out of the indirect medical education payments. So one would suspect, at least from a policy perspective, that the intent was to keep them as distinct funding streams.

I would like to reinforce one of Lewin's observations regarding research. Issues relating to intellectual property rights, conflict of interest, protection of human subjects, privacy considerations, and an array of science policy issues have increased in number and complexity. Those topics currently are being dealt with in separate contexts. I think public policymakers should step back, note how they are intertwined, and consider the consequences of any proposed changes. Some proposed interventions that would excessively constrain access to historic databases and constrain incentives may be adverse to research down the road.

Some improvements have been made in funding new technology. Medicare now has a mechanism for both outpatient and inpatient care that permits pass-through of the costs of new devices and drugs for a limited period of time. It will be important to monitor the impact of those changes.

Finally, I would like to join those who have observed that academic medical centers have a large stake in reducing the ranks of the uninsured. Significant percentages of patients at some of the major teaching hospitals are covered by Medicaid or are uninsured. If we are fortunate enough to solve or substantially address the uninsured problem, we are going to have another: such a happy occurrence could disrupt patient flows to many teaching hospitals. That is not, of course, reason to avoid seeking aggressive solutions to the first problem. But it is a likely consequence that we need to think through and be prepared to deal with.

The purpose of the third section of the meeting is to deal with practical public policy options. Academic medical centers, teaching hospitals, and medical schools are generally viewed as inefficient. While I am not sure we know how to measure efficiency in many instances, I would agree with that opinion. I am not sure, however, that they are any more inefficient than other sectors of the health care system or academia. Furthermore, one should remember that patient care, education, and research are interrelated. Because of that, teaching hospitals would be costly even if they operated with complete efficiency; the question is how to cover the additional costs. Historically, at least for clinically related activities, those costs have been paid either by explicit payment mechanisms in Medicare and some Medicaid programs or by implicit mechanisms (higher charges) in the private sector. I believe that the Medicare model is a good model of how to cover such real, important, and nonstandard costs. We have almost twenty years of experience with the Medicare model: we know its faults, its shortcomings, and its strengths. In fact, many of the problems that people have identified in terms of perverse incentives have been dealt with to some degree through legislation and regulation.

We may yet have an opportunity to look at an all-payer system based on the Medicare model to gather funds from the entire delivery system. Gail Wilensky mentioned the higher-than-justified payments for indirect medical education provided through Medicare. An all-payer system would have the potential additional benefit of reducing the level of some of the current funding provided by Medicare.

I know that many people do not believe that it is practical or politically feasible to continue to use and expand the Medicare models of support for direct and indirect medical education. But I am not sure that doing so is any less practical and politically feasible than implementing many of the alternatives that have been proposed in the debate, which has continued for more than a decade. So I would urge us all to make sure that an all-payer system is on the list of policy options.

COMMENT BY
Kenneth I. Shine

Before making my comments, I would like to identify several potential conflicts of interest. The Robert Wood Johnson Foundation has provided funding to the Institute of Medicine (IOM) to undertake four to six studies over the next three years on the economic, health, and social consequences of the lack of health insurance that exists among a large number of Americans. The IOM also is completing plans for a project on the nursing work force and in late 2001 will initiate a two-year study on the future of academic health centers.

I believe that the number of medical schools is more likely to increase than decrease. The poor distribution of medical schools is not new. Several states with rapidly growing populations, particularly of Hispanics—

including California, Florida, and Texas—want improved access of their residents to medical education. Florida already is committed to one additional school. In many of these states, the pressure will be enormous to increase the number of students at existing schools, the number of schools, or both.

Retaining the cap on the number of graduate medical education (GME) positions is essential to increasing educational opportunities for U.S. citizens. If the number of well-trained American students competing for the currently fixed number of GME positions were to increase, the number of foreign medical graduates coming to train in the United States would diminish without any external regulation. An increase in the number of GME slots would be counterproductive because it would add to the potential oversupply of U.S. physicians.

If public policy is to offer enduring support to academic medical centers, the centers must do more to strengthen themselves. Although David Blumenthal has emphasized the role of location as a major determinant of the success of AMCs, I believe that good management is vital. The successful program that Spike Foreman describes in the Bronx is testimony not so much to location as to his management skills. Despite his concerns about his institution's balance sheet, he knows how to organize such programs and he manages them well. Unfortunately, academic health centers at least until recently have not valued management training, experience, and expertise. The leaders of AMCs often have been successful in research or patient care but poorly prepared to manage large, complex organizations. Not only should hospital boards value managers and management, but public and private policy should better prepare individuals to manage through formal and informal educational programs.

While some academic medical centers have had serious financial problems, many schools are doing very well. Not all of AMCs' problems have resulted from bad management, but one cannot understand the debacle of the Allegheny Health Center without recognizing the role of managerial blunders spread over several years. Misconceived merger strategies account for other failures; flaws included both a defective vision for the institution and a failure to understand fundamental problems of faculty culture.

Who actually owns AMCs remains a conundrum. The trustees? Management? The faculty? The community? Absence of an understanding of who is in charge obstructs effective collaboration among the components and hobbles rational attempts to formulate a mission, goals, objectives, and strategies.

A fundamental problem of AMCs regarding costs arises out of multitasking. I agree with Joseph Newhouse's suggestion that the Financial Accounting Standards Board try to fashion uniform accounting standards for academic medical centers. However, faculty members often provide clinical care, teach, and do clinical research simultaneously. I would applaud an effort to rationally allocate costs among those functions, but success in such an effort is not ensured.

While academic health centers continue to provide complex care, applying the latest in medical technology, it is worth noting that the increase in the cost of devices and pharmaceuticals has caused expenditures for devices and drugs to exceed payments to hospitals in several major metropolitan areas. As ambulatory care continues to expand and noninvasive ambulatory surgical procedures increase, hospitals may be competing for a decreasing proportion of the health care dollar. In such an environment, it is going to be harder to make a case for the special role of the hospital. At the same time, medical education continues to focus strongly on inpatient care; although education in ambulatory care has improved, it still represents a small portion of the curriculum in most medical schools. In order to bring education in ambulatory care up to the level of the intense educational experience in inpatient care, there will have to be substantially increased emphasis on teaching students how to participate in decisionmaking, to use *systems* of care, and to engage in an ongoing effort to improve quality of care.

Regarding health science research, I strongly support efforts to reexamine the requirement that institutions receiving extramural research grants share part of the research costs. Cost sharing emerged as individual investigators and the National Institutes of Health began to find ways to increase the proportion of funds available to investigators and decrease the proportion allocated to indirect costs, which went to institutions. Administrative costs were capped at 26 percent; that policy, coupled with other efforts to control indirect expenditures, progressively increased the pressure on institutions. Each dollar of extramural research support now requires an estimated 20 to 25 cents of direct institutional research support.

While some cost sharing can be defended, the amount requires careful study. Most universities operate under provisions for indirect costs described by a federal policy called A21, which makes no allowance for direct costs associated with starting new programs; in contrast, industrial contractors and other organizations operate under A122, which authorizes use of part of a grant to support the costs of program initiation. Providing funds directly to AMCs to support the start-up of new research projects, including costs for equipment and some salary support, merits serious consideration. Such grants should be based on a peer review process to avoid some of the difficulties associated with the basic group research support plans that were phased out in the 1980s.

Despite the future importance of education in ambulatory care, Medicare funds to support graduate medical education now go to the hospital in most academic health centers. I believe that a significant portion of those funds should be applied specifically to the support of educational and patient care efforts in the ambulatory arena; in addition, it would be far better if those funds were transferred to and managed by faculty practice plans. Ambulatory facilities currently are run by hospitals in many institutions, creating a perverse incentive to allocate inpatient costs to ambulatory units. As a result, inpatient activity appears to be financially stable and outpatient activity shows considerable deficits.

Moreover, teaching and patient care in the ambulatory arena are not coupled with financial incentives for the faculty to operate efficiently and effectively. Providing GME funds to the faculty practice plans with the requirement that they manage ambulatory services independently would clearly identify lines of responsibility and cost centers. If the hospital is to provide funds for the ambulatory arena, they would be clearly identified as a contribution to the outpatient cost centers. Gradually shifting GME funds to the ambulatory arena, beginning with 10 percent and rising to one-third over the next five years, would rationalize education and patient care and better define responsibility.

Information systems designed for health care systems continue to be extremely expensive and remarkably ineffective. There is no common language and no requirement for connectivity among information systems, even within departments and among the various components of an AMC; connectivity, not surprisingly, is poor. Systems designed for performing administrative tasks often are used to analyze quality of care. A major public policy initiative in this area is required. Medicare, for example, could authorize use of funds for hardware and software investments in information systems, provided they met standards for content, used a common language, and were connected to other units within the medical center. Building a national infrastructure for information systems and informatics in health care is one of the major challenges for this decade.

I strongly support efforts to invest in research on education and the educational process. Both have been neglected. We need new paradigms for education that involve various health professionals—nursing students, medical students, pharmacists, and others—solving problems together in various settings. Those groups need to understand the culture of each other's profession as well as how the health care system works and how to solve problems within the system. Medical education needs to prepare practitioners for change and for a continual effort to improve quality of care. A federal investment in medical education would educate not only students, but also faculty members, few of whom now understand those principles.

New policies to finance care for the indigent deserve high priority. A range of experiments such as the one reported by Spencer Foreman illustrate what can be done, and they should be encouraged. Any thoughtful observer of the U.S. health care system understands that the United States desperately needs universal health insurance coverage, but only marginal change can be expected in the near future. Although the demand for indigent care now imposes a heavy burden on many medical centers, extension of coverage might actually reduce occupancy of medical centers if newly insured patients elect to receive care elsewhere.

Academic health centers are large and complex; consequently, complying with the proliferation of occupational, environmental, administrative, and other rules and regulations can be particularly costly for them. While some regulations are essential for health and safety, simplification to clarify the relationships among regulations from multiple agencies and to eliminate conflicting policies is both possible and desirable.

Finally, increased investment in health science research is likely to produce revolutionary and unpredictable change. Plans to double the NIH budget are exciting and deserve support; however, the notion to double occurred when growth of health care costs was relatively low. Cost growth now has begun to accelerate, and it is likely to increase substantially over the next several years, driven by the cost of new medical devices and pharmaceuticals. Rising costs could well produce a backlash. Academic health centers will have an increasing responsibility to carefully study technology transfer, to evaluate the marginal value of new technologies, and to ensure that rising costs do not become unaffordable. If academic medical centers can perform those and other functions well, they will provide a vital service to society, ultimately—and not incidentally—strengthening society's commitment to academic health centers.

COMMENT BY
Gail Wilensky

I do not disagree with Lawrence Lewin's general theme, which is that the role of academic medical centers is to educate the health care work force, carry out basic and clinical research, and provide advanced specialty care and care for uninsured and underserved patients. However, I would like to put the role of academic medical centers in a somewhat different context.

Let me start with care for the uninsured and uncompensated care. Historically, academic health centers have played an important role in providing care for the indigent; Lewin argues that unless or until health insurance coverage is universal, that role will remain important. There is some truth to that point. As long as many people lack health insurance coverage, academic health centers, as well as public hospitals, will remain providers of last resort. Although the number of people without health insurance could decline substantially, even without a system of universal coverage, it is unlikely to do so.

More generally, I think that it is important to realize that saying "indigent care" is not sufficient justification for cross-subsidies until such time as universal health insurance becomes a reality. The question is whether care for the uninsured and uncompensated care justify the full extent of current cross-subsidies. That question is not a quibble. Several strategies, which may or may not come to fruition, hold considerable promise for extending health coverage to low-income and working uninsured populations.

Whether anything comes of those proposals remains to be seen, but if the proportion of the population without health insurance coverage were to fall from 16 percent to a third of that—that is, if 95 percent of the population were insured—then the responsibilities of academic health centers would be seen in a different light. In particular, the case for maintaining the current level of cross-subsidies within AMCs would be difficult to justify. Substantial reduction in the uninsured population is much more likely than universal availability of health care, which I think is unlikely in my lifetime for a lot of reasons, not the least of which is that the transfer of power to government that would be necessary to achieve it is unlikely to occur.

Aside from the aggregate amount of care provided, it is frustrating to try to defend the reasonableness of a strategy to provide substantial cross-subsidies for care for the uninsured because cross-subsidies are such a terribly clumsy mechanism for financing that care. While it is true that academic health centers on average have provided a substantial amount of uncompensated care, not all have done so and many other institutions also provide a considerable amount. It is not very hard to understand why. How much uncompensated care an institution is called on to provide depends more on where it is located than on the disposition of the institution's managers.

Lewin also mentioned that the Balanced Budget Act of 1997 had a chilling effect on uninsured care because it reduced disproportionate share hospital (DSH) payments. As chair of MedPAC, I probably look at that issue with a slightly jaundiced view. Medicare DSH dollars do not compensate for uncovered Medicare costs, but instead provide funding for general uncompensated care. The DSH program has been an even clumsier way of paying for uninsured care than the cross-subsidies embedded in graduate medical education (GME) payments because of the peculiar rules governing the distribution of DSH funds between urban and rural hospitals and because of the way that the low-income population has been defined for the purpose of disbursing DSH monies. Some of these problems were corrected by the Benefit Improvement and Protection Act legislation passed in December 2000.

Medicaid DSH transfers involve substantially more money than do Medicare DSH transfers, and Medicaid is even more poorly designed to provide funding for the uninsured. The "creative financing" by states that I observed as administrator of the Health Care Financing Administration is at least as egregious today. Voluntary donations and provider taxes have been replaced by payment claims that exceed actual spending for Medicaid. Congress is now trying to curb that practice with so-called upper-payment limits.

Medicaid DSH payments are substantial—roughly $8.2 billion in 2000—but it is difficult to assess how DSH money is spent. Whether it is providing care for the uninsured or even going to health care is unclear. Anyone who is worried about the problems of the uninsured should regard DSH payments as a very unsatisfactory response.

Let me be clear. As much as I dislike DSH payments and other untargeted cross-subsidies as a way to respond to the problem of caring for the uninsured and uncompensated care, I recognize that it is necessary to be careful about the order in which corrections are made. A better mechanism must be in place before these clumsy cross-subsidies are eliminated.

In short, it is important to recognize that the health care needs of the uninsured must be financed. It is equally important to recognize that cross-subsidies and DSH payments are bad ways to do so. In addition, of course, many academic health institutions may not be the best places for the uninsured to receive most of their primary and secondary care. Some institutions have developed efficient, well-coordinated primary care facilities; others are less desirable but provide care if no other institution will do so. But in general advanced tertiary medical care providers should not be called on to provide primary care for large populations.

It may make some sense for academic medical centers to provide primary care because they train physicians and physicians need to learn to provide primary and secondary care. But in those instances it is less clear who ought to pay, particularly if that care could be provided more efficiently in another setting. That, certainly, is a legitimate question for public policy.

That academic medical centers should be in the forefront of clinical and biomedical research is clear. They have played an important part in this arena, supporting the leading role that the United States has played in biomedical science in general and in such specific endeavors as the human genome project. But, like it or not, the country is moving from a world of implicit cross-subsidies into a world of explicit financing. That means that funding clinical and biomedical research that nobody is knowingly willing to pay for is going to become more and more difficult. Whether one approves of that shift—and I do—it is a political fact of life. I sympathize with academic health centers that have to respond to the match requirement for NIH funding. Along with Lewin, I think it is time to modify that requirement—but not to eliminate it. However, rules that worked in a world with large cross-subsidies will not work in a world in which there is primary reliance on explicit financing.

I agree that academic medical centers are—and should be—places where sophisticated care is provided and where technological innovation ensures that procedures and devices are state of the art. MedPAC and ProPAC before it have long agreed that academic health centers incur additional costs because they provide sophisticated, state-of-the-art care with specialized personnel on site or on call all of the time. Those costs are the rationale for indirect medical education payments. I agree with this policy, which leads to the last issue, that of how to deal with graduate medical education. MedPAC has concluded that the distinction between direct and indirect medical education that began in the 1980s is not helpful. The kind of training received in residency is generalized training that stays with the person who has been trained; according to standard economic theory, the student bears the costs for such training. Rather than get into a fight about whether GME is being restructured to save money, MedPAC recommended that Medicare continue to provide the amounts now being spent for direct and indirect education to institutions to help compensate for the additional patient care costs even though it appears that the combined payments are above an empirically justified level. But MedPAC did not recommend a change in the structure of payments starting in 1999.

Many people think that direct training costs are borne by the institutions; they propose other ways to handle GME. An all-payer system—a charge levied on all payers to support graduate medical education—is one such proposal. To me, an all-payer system is simply a tax, and a hidden or implicit one at that. If the government believes that it is a public responsibility to support GME, reimbursement for these costs should go through the appropriations process. The federal government has a long history of providing grants, loans, and subsidies to individuals to make sure that they have an opportunity to pursue the American dream, using education as a vehicle for the redistribution of income. That practice applies to ensuring talented youngsters' access to the medical profession, including nursing—but it justifies grants to individuals, not to institutions.

The nursing problem is just beginning to get the attention that it merits. If there is a nursing shortage that will not be sorted out over time, public policy should focus on reducing the cost of training to the trainee. The problem is not a shortage of training slots; it results, at least in part, from the reality that women now have options that were not available before—including the option to become a doctor instead of a nurse. The attempt of the nursing profession to eliminate training programs for individuals without a bachelor's or master's degree may not have been very helpful; people with two years of training can perform many nursing tasks. The mix of health workers is likely to change in the future. Nurses' wages probably will have to increase, at least for those doing advanced nursing. That is how a market economy responds to labor shortages.

General Discussion

Herbert Pardes seconded the emphasis a number of speakers had placed on the high cost of information technology and of its importance in both clinical care and education. He also returned to the question raised in previous sessions of the desirability of allowing the bottom 25 percent of AMCs to close down. He distinguished a reduction in the number of hospitals from a reduction in the number of medical schools. Currently, about 16,000 students finish U.S. medical schools each year, but 25,000 residencies are available. Reducing the number of residencies is very different from reducing the number of schools. If the number of schools is reduced without lowering the number of residencies, the result will be simply more entry opportunities for foreign medical graduates.

Kathy Buto noted that it is important to keep a broad perspective when proposing Medicare reforms to address the problems facing academic medical centers. For example, she mentioned that changes such as modifications in the way diagnosis related groups (DRG) pass-through provisions reimburse new technologies contribute to significant and potentially harmful biases toward capital-intensive procedures. If the same increase in payments was provided through an addition to the annual general update factor for DRG payments, hospitals would be better able to decide what investments address their needs best.

Lawrence Lewin agreed that distortions can arise from procedure-linked adjustments but noted that for some of the new procedures, particularly those based on radiation, some targeted adjustments also were necessary.

References

Commonwealth Fund Task Force on Academic Health Centers. 1997. *Leveling the Playing Field: Financing the Missions of Academic Health Centers.* New York: Commonwealth Fund.

Coughlin, T., L. Ku, and J. Kim. 2000. *Reforming the Medicaid Disproportionate Share Hospital Program in the 1990s.* Discussion Paper 99–14. Washington: The Urban Institute.

Davis, K., C. Schoen, and S. Schoenbaum. 2000. "A 2020 Vision for American Health Care." *Archives of Internal Medicine* 160 (December 11/25).

Ghadebo, A. L., and U. E. Reinhardt. 2001. "Economists on Academic Medicine: Elephants in a Porcelain Shop?" *Health Affairs* 20 (2).

Health Resources and Services Administration, U.S. Department of Health and Human Services. 2001. *Hard Numbers, Hard Choices.*

Kahn, C. N., III, and R. F. Pollack. 2001. "Strange Bedfellows: Consensus for Reform." *Health Affairs* 20 (1).

Kaiser Commission on Medicaid and the Uninsured. 2001. *The Medicaid Program at a Glance.* Washington: The Henry J. Kaiser Family Foundation.

Ku, L., and T. Coughlin. 1995. "Medicaid Disproportionate Share and Other Special Financing Programs." *Health Care Financing Review* 16 (3).

Mann, Joyce M., and others. 1997. "A Profile of Uncompensated Hospital Care, 1983–1995." *Health Affairs* 16 (4).

Medicare Payment Advisory Commission. 2001. *Report to the Congress: Medicare's Payment Policy.*

Meyer, G., and D. Blumenthal. 1996. *The Initial Effects of TennCare on Academic Health Centers.* New York: The Commonwealth Fund.

Shortliffe, E. H. 2000. "Networking Health: Learning from Others, Taking the Lead." *Health Affairs* 19 (6).

Contributors

Henry J. Aaron
Brookings Institution

David Blumenthal
Institute for Health Policy, Massachusetts General Hospital

Spencer Foreman
Montefiore Medical Center

Nancy M. Kane
Harvard School of Public Health

Edward Miller
Johns Hopkins University School of Medicine

Ralph Muller
University of Chicago Hospitals and Health System

James Robinson
School of Public Health, University of California, Berkeley

James Reuter
Institute for Health Care Research Policy, Georgetown University

Peter Van Etten
Juvenile Diabetes Foundation

Index

AAMC. *See* Association of American
  Medical Colleges
Aaron, Henry, 45, 71
Academic medical centers (AMCs):
  bond-rating agencies, 7, 13; clinical
  trials, 59; competition and, 45–46,
  50, 51, 62, 71; divestiture, 49, 56,
  59, 61, 100; faculty and personnel,
  7, 34, 36, 43, 45, 46, 63, 79, 82,
  93; high-, medium-, and low-
  performance groups, 26–31, 35, 36,
  37, 41, 44, 45; renewal of, 35–36,
  37, 38; technology and research,
  43, 50–51, 53. *See also* Hospitals;
  Johns Hopkins Medicine; Medical
  and nursing schools; Montefiore
  Medical Center; Research
Academic medical centers (AMCs)—
  administration and management:
  accounting issues, 71, 81; ambulatory facilities or physician practices,
  44; analysis of financial health, 14–
  31, 42, 58; availability of financial
  data, 21–22; as businesses, 4, 45,
  63; cost management, 32; effects of
  poor administration, 8, 34, 37;
  management of Medicare funds, 94;
  Massachusetts community hospitals, 45; past and present view of,
  55–56; reporting practices, 15, 18–

20, 36, 39, 40, 41, 46; response to
  worsening financial environment,
  6–10; understanding of cross-
  subsidies, 42; "who is in charge,"
  92–93
Academic medical centers (AMCs)—
  definition and organization:
  activities and products, 50, 62,
  96; complexity of, 14–15, 62, 75–
  76; definition, 1–2; integrated
  delivery systems, 61–62, 71;
  provision of care, 76, 77, 78, 83–
  87, 90, 96–97, 98–99; research
  mission, 56, 57–60, 62–63, 70, 81;
  specialty clinical services, 59–60;
  types of, 23
Academic medical centers (AMCs)—
  financial issues: appropriation of
  innovation in medicine, 57–60;
  challenges to financial stability, 49–
  50; financial status and history, 2–
  4, 41; income and investments, 20,
  36, 37–38, 40, 44, 46, 56, 71;
  margins and profitability, 37, 43,
  85, 93; rules and regulations, 95;
  spending, 45; strategies for, 8–11,
  45–46, 62–63
Academic Medicine, 89
Accreditation Council for Graduate
  Medical Education, 89

Agency for Healthcare Research and
   Quality, 86
AHA. *See* American Hospital
   Association
Albert Einstein College of
   Medicine, 64
Allegheny Health, Education, and
   Research Foundation (AHERF), 7,
   15, 56, 92
AMCs. *See* Academic medical centers
American Hospital Association
   (AHA), 9, 21, 22, 34, 77
American Telephone and Telegraph
   (ATT), 52
Association of American Medical
   Colleges (AAMC): data provided,
   9, 23; financial state of academic
   medicine, 34, 39; graduate medical
   education, 89; mission accounting
   work, 81; surveys, 21, 22
ATT. *See* American Telephone and
   Telegraph

Balanced Budget Act of 1997 (BBA):
   disproportionate share hospital
   payments, 84, 97; effects on
   hospitals, 11, 32, 35, 76; freeze on
   cuts, 13; Medicare and Medicaid
   payments, 5, 9
Balanced Budget Refinement Act of
   1999, 11
Baylor University, 7
BBA. *See* Balanced Budget Act
   of 1997
Benefit Improvement and Protection
   Act of 2000, 97
Beth Israel Deaconess Medical Center
   (BIDMC), 15, 18
BIDMC. *See* Beth Israel Deaconess
   Medical Center
Biles, Brian, 45
Blumenthal, David, 61–63, 72, 92

Boston (MA), 61
Bronx (NY), 64, 66, 92
Buto, Kathy, 100

California, 42, 91–92
CareGroup. *See* Harvard University
Center for Healthcare Industry
   Performance Studies (CHIPS),
   26, 32
Centers for Medicare and Medicaid
   Services (CMS). See Health Care
   Financing Administration (HCFA)
Charitable organizations, 10, 21
Charleston Area Medical Center,
   30–31
CHIPS. *See* Center for Healthcare
   Industry Performance Studies
Clinical trials. *See* Research
Clinton, Bill, 37
Clinton Health Plan, 77
Commonwealth Fund, 77
Commonwealth Task Force on
   Academic Health Centers, 38–39
Community medicine, 79
Computers. *See* Technology
Congressional Budget Office, 84
Congress, U.S., 77, 85
Connecticut, 44
COTH. *See* Council of Teaching
   Hospitals
Council of Teaching Hospitals
   (COTH), 23

Dartmouth University, 18
Department of Health and Human
   Services (DHHS), 85
Detroit Medical Center, 31
DHHS. *See* Department of Health and
   Human Services
Diagnosis related group (DRG). *See*
   Medicare
Dickler, Robert, 45, 88–91

Disproportionate share hospital (DSH). *See* Medicare
Divestiture. *See* Academic Medical Centers
Dobson, Allen, 44, 70
DRG (diagnosis related group). *See* Medicare
Drucker, Peter, 62
DSH (disproportionate share hospital). *See* Medicare
Duke University, 7

Economic theory of innovation, 50
Endowments, 36, 40, 44, 71
Ernst and Young, 42

Families U.S.A., 77
FASB. *See* Financial Accounting Standards Board
Financial Accounting Standards Board (FASB), 71, 93
Financial issues: AMC financial analyses, 25–31; definitions, 30; financial equilibrium, 35; financial reports, 35; renewal of physical and human capital, 35–36; standardized accounting methods, 71; trends, 32–33. *See also* Academic medical centers—financial issues
Florida, 91–92
Foreman, Spencer, 43, 64–67, 71, 92, 95

Gatorade, 82
Georgetown University, 39
George Washington University, 1
GME (graduate medical education). *See* Medical and nursing schools
Government, federal and state: development of standards, 87; funding of health research and training, 4, 84–85, 99; grants, 51, 53, 57; new policies, 11; purchaser of AMC services, 72, 75–76; State Children's Health Insurance Program, 85; venture capital fund, 82–83
Graduate medical education (GME). *See* Medical and nursing schools
Grants: cost-sharing, 81–82, 93–94; National Institutes of Health, 57, 79; research grants, 51, 53, 57, 81

Harvard University: CareGroup, 7, 14–15, 16–17, 56; clinical practice and hospital, 1; clinical trials, 63
HCFA. *See* Health Care Financing Administration
Health Affairs, 8–9, 41
Healthcare Financial Management Association, 22 Health Care Financing Administration (HCFA): excess capacity, 45; prospective payments, 5; reforms by, 86; study of financial state of academic medicine, 34; timeliness of financial reporting, 22
Health Insurance Association of America, 77
Health Insurance Plan of New York, 66
Health maintenance organizations (HMOs), 35, 37
Health Security Act, 37
Hellman, Samuel, 70
HMOs. *See* Health maintenance organizations
Hospital of the University of Pennsylvania, 18, 30, 31
Hospitals: administration, 44–45; closures of, 10, 45; distributed networks, 37; excess capacity, 45; failure of, 44; insurance effects, 3; inpatient and outpatient services,

42, 94; losses, 37; Medicare and, 5, 94; mergers, 7–8; occupancy rates, 3, 5–6, 7; pharmaceutical costs, 35; profitability, 41; public, 78; quality and variety of health services, 2–3; ratings, 56; regional variations, 23–25; revenue and financial issues, 2, 5–7, 9, 11, 36; surplus of hospital beds, 10; teaching and university hospitals, 36, 50, 85, 90–91. *See also* Academic medical centers
Human genome project, 83

IDS. *See* Integrated delivery systems
Informatics and information, 87, 94–95. *See also* Technology
Innovation, 51-53, 54-56. *See also* Research; Technology
Institute of Medicine (IOM), 91
Insurance: bond insurance, 7; commercial insurers, 44; cost of care and, 37, 78; effects on hospital use, 3; financing care for the indigent, 76, 77, 95; Medicaid and Medicare, 5; provider-owned plans, 42; uninsured people, 6, 10, 91; universal, 77, 85–86, 95, 96. *See also* Health maintenance organizations; Managed care; Medicaid; Medicare; Subsidies
Integrated delivery systems (IDS), 61–62, 71
Intellectual property, 51–52
Internal Revenue Service (IRS) Form 990, 15, 21, 22
Internet. *See* Technology
Investments. *See* Academic medical centers
IOM. *See* Institute of Medicine
IRS. *See* Internal Revenue Service

Johns Hopkins Medicine, 7, 67–70

Kane, Nancy M., 13–46, 72, 85

Lewin, Lawrence, 44, 70–71, 75–100

Managed care, 3, 5, 67, 83
Mary Hitchcock Medical Center (MHMC), 18
Massachusetts, 33, 44, 45
Massachusetts General Hospital, 8
MCR. *See* Medicare Cost Reports
Medicaid: contracts with managed care organizations, 5; disproportionate share hospital (DSH) reimbursements, 89–90, 97; eligibility for, 85; payments by, 9, 36, 42, 44, 84, 86
Medical and nursing schools: course of study, 2, 89, 93; education and educational problems, 78–81; faculty, 81; financial support of medical education, 86, 89, 95, 99; graduate medical education positions, 92, 99; indigent care and, 83; Medicare payments for, 83–84; need for, 77–78; number of medical and nursing students, 88–89, 99; numbers of, 77, 88, 91–92; research into, 95; residencies, 100; revenue flows, 2, 3–4. *See also* Academic medical centers
Medical science, 2, 3*f*
Medicare: computer investments, 94–95; cost of care and, 37; cost reports, 15; diagnosis related group (DRG) payments, 83, 85, 86, 100; disproportionate share hospital; eimbursements, 76, 78, 84, 89–90, 97; hospitals, 84; margins, 38, 85; medical education, 76, 83–84, 89, 91, 94, 99; Medicare+Choice, 86; payments by, 2, 5, 8, 9, 11, 36, 44, 76; pharmaceutical costs, 35;

reform of, 11; reimbursement for preventative medicine, 85; uniform billing form, 87

Medicare Cost Reports (MCR), 21, 26

Medicare Payment Advisory Commission (MedPAC): Medicare data, 37, 76, 85; support of graduate medical education, 86, 89; view of academic medical centers, 34, 41, 98–99; view of hospitals, 9

Meharry Medical College, 61

Memphis (TN), 61

MHMC. *See* Mary Hitchcock Medical Center

Miller, Edward, 67–70

Mind-Body Institute, 15

Montefiore Medical Center, 64–67, 72

Moody's, 56

Muller, Ralph, 34–38, 43

National Institutes of Health (NIH): budget, 95; cost-sharing, 70, 98, 93; funding of research, 57, 79, 81; grants to Johns Hopkins Medicine, 69–70; technology transfer, 82–83

Newhouse, Joseph, 71, 93

New York, 44

NIH. *See* National Institutes of Health

Nonprofit organizations, 22, 56

Nursing schools. *See* Medical and nursing schools

Pardes, Herbert, 43, 72, 100

Partners Healthcare System, 8

Penn State. *See* Pennsylvania State

Pennsylvania, 44

Pennsylvania State (Penn State), 56

Peter Bent Brigham Hospital (Boston, MA), 8

Pharmaceuticals and pharmaceutical companies: business strategy, 62; clinical trials, 59; cost of, 35, 43; as integrated organizations, 54; role of companies, 43

Philanthropic giving, 71, 85

Physicians and physician practices: community doctors, 46; diversity and distribution, 89; foreign, 92; interests of patients, 8; purchase of, 8. *See also* Medical and nursing schools

Policies and policy reforms: alleviating AMC financial distress, 33–34, 35; new technology, 90; nursing, 80; reductions of Medicaid/Medicare payments, 36–37

Reischauer, Robert, 44, 45

Reuter, James, 38–40

Religious organizations, 10

Research: academic medical centers, 98; appropriation of economic benefits, 54–56; biotechnology and medical devices, 58; clinical trials, 59; computers and, 87; cost-sharing, 93–94; disease causes and treatment, 79; educational methods, 80; funding and costs, 51, 53, 69, 70, 93, 98; laboratory research excluding biotechnology, 57–58; in the life sciences, 81–83; institutional research support, 93; patent protection, 52, 53; policy issues, 90; salary caps, 82. *See also* Innovation; Technology

Reuter, James, 44, 45

Robert Wood Johnson Foundation, 77, 91

Robinson, James C., 49–72

S&P. *See* Standard & Poor's

SCHIP. *See* State Children's Health
Insurance Program
SEC. *See* Securities and Exchange
Commission
Securities and Exchange Commission
(SEC), 22
Shine, Kenneth, 43, 44–45, 70, 91–96
Standard & Poor's (S&P), 13–14, 56
Stanford University, 7, 56
State Children's Health Insurance
Program (SCHIP), 85, 86
Statistical analysis, 35
"Strange Bedfellows Proposal," 77
Subsidies: cross-subsidies, 41, 44, 53,
58, 78, 96–97, 98; loss of, 42; to
faculty practices, 43; University of
California, 42

Tax issues, 71
Technology: academic medical centers
and, 43, 95; compatibility, 52;
computer-based systems of learning, 80; conversion to, 10; effects
on hospital stays, 2, 3; effects on
profitability, 43; integrated
companies, 55; Internet, 86;
medical devices, 85; technology
transfer, 82–83; telecommunications, 87–88; venture capital fund,
82–83. *See also* Innovation;
Research

Texas, 91–92
2020 Vision for American Health
Care, 77, 85

UHC. *See* University Health Care
Consortium
Universities: costs, 93–94; endow-
ments, 36; research, 58; spending
rules, 36; tenure system, 70–71;
university hospitals, 50, 56
University Health Care Consortium
(UHC), 81
University HealthSystem Consortium,
34, 39, 42
University of California, 7, 42, 56
University of Florida, 82
University of Pennsylvania, 7, 8,
18, 56
University of Pittsburgh Medical
Center (UPMC), 19
UPMC. *See* University of Pittsburgh
Medical Center

Vanderbilt Medical Center, 61
Van Etten, Peter, 40–42, 70, 71, 81
Vladeck, Bruce, 34, 42–43, 71–72

Washington University, 7
Wilensky, Gail, 89, 91, 96–99